W9-DGX-520

the BUSINESS *of* MASSAGE

The Complete Guide to Establishing Your Massage Career

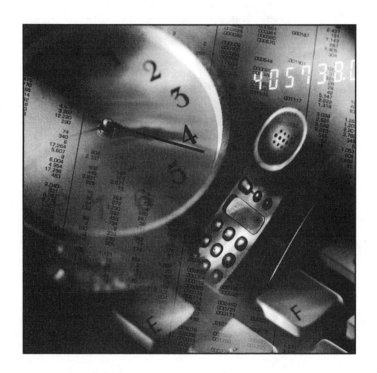

A publication written by and for practitioners
of the massage therapy profession

Published by
American Massage Therapy Association®

820 Davis Street, Suite 100
Evanston, IL 60201-4444
Phone (847) 864-0123   Fax (847) 864-1178
www.amtamassage.org

Published by: American Massage Therapy Association
820 Davis Street, Suite 100
Evanston, IL 60201-4444
847-864-0123
www.amtamassage.org

©2002

DEVELOPMENT TEAM

Project Management: Simon & Kolz Publishing, Dubuque, Iowa
Textbook Development: Jean Pascual, Words Unleashed, Galena, Illinois
Instructor Guide Development: Maija Rothenberg, Balagot Communications, Inc., Chicago, Illinois
Book Design and Layout: Kelly Fassbinder, Imagine Design, Dubuque, Iowa

All rights reserved.
No part of this publication may be reproduced, stored in a retrieval system, or transmitted, in any form or by any means whether electronic, mechanical, photocopying, recording or otherwise, without the prior written permission of the publisher (AMTA).

This publication is intended to provide general guidance and information and is not meant to be a substitute for professional legal, financial, or tax advice, which should be obtained through consultation with appropriate professionals in your state. The information contained herein is provided "as is" and AMTA makes no representation or warranty that the information will be timely or error free. All names of companies, persons, and entities are fictitious unless otherwise noted. Please direct any comments, questions, or suggestions regarding this book to AMTA, *The Business of Massage*, at the address above.

ISBN: 1-929947-06-2

TABLE *of* CONTENTS

Preface and Acknowledgements

Congratulations on preparing to enter the profession of massage! *The Business of Massage* was written to help you learn the business basics you will need to operate your practice. The content of this book was based largely on the *American Massage Therapy Association Massage Therapy Career Guide* series of business manuals. When that series was developed by and for Professional members of the American Massage Therapy Association, members recommended that similar content be made available in textbook format for the benefit of students who will be starting their own practices as massage therapists.

The business basics found in this book—how to find a job, how to start your own business, how to do the financial, administrative, and marketing functions to run a healthy business—are applicable to just about any small business. But what makes this book essential for you, the massage therapy student, is that its content is tailored to your needs as a professional.

Massage therapists are unique from other professionals in many ways. You must be competent in your understanding and behavior with regard to ethical issues specific to the practice of massage. You must be knowledgeable of the scope and standards of practice in the profession, as well as the regulations that will affect you in the state or province in which you practice. You must make decisions regarding business policies about whether to discount your services, whether to accept tips, and whether to accept third-party reimbursement (insurance) clients. You also are in a unique position to appeal to consumers whose perception of massage is increasingly more positive than it was in the past.

You will find that the book allows you to gain a perspective on the profession as a whole (in chapter 1) before you are asked to decide how you want to begin your professional career. Chapter 2 helps you start to create the outline of your business plan, which is applicable to you whether you decide to work as an employee or start your own business. Throughout chapters 3 through 6, you will add more details to the framework of your business plan in the areas of setting up your office and practice room, creating recordkeeping systems, planning your daily routine, and establishing policies that support your therapeutic relationship with clients. By chapter 7, in which you will learn marketing strategies and tactics, you will have an understanding of who your clients probably will be and how you will attract them to your business. The final chapter presents food for thought about what it means to be a professional massage therapist. It discusses the benefits of involvement in a professional association, the need for continuing education, and the growing opportunities to become involved in massage research.

Many of the business tools illustrated in the textbook are available as forms for use in your own practice. Wherever you see *The Business of Massage* logo in the corner of an illustration, it means that this tool or form is contained in *The Business Forms Packet* from which you may reproduce copies for your own use.

Because experienced massage therapists and educators developed this book, it is filled with *Shared Wisdom* notes—advice and counsel that reflects the personal experiences of many individual practitioners. It is into this unique body of wisdom that experienced massage therapists invite you, and it is their hope that this book will be one of the tools that can aid you on your way to full participation in the profession.

IN GRATEFUL ACKNOWLEDGEMENT

The American Massage Therapy Association would like to thank the many individuals who generously shared their time, knowledge, and learning materials in the creation of this book. Special thanks go to Barry Antoniow for permitting liberal use of content from *Business Success Handbook*, which he wrote for use with his own students at, first, the Professional Institute of Massage Therapy, Saskatchewan, and now at Kiné-Concept Institute Maritimes, New Brunswick. Special appreciation also goes to Carole Ostendorf, PhD, executive director of the Commission on Massage Therapy Accreditation (COMTA), for ensuring that the content of this book reflects the competencies required of accredited schools of massage therapy and bodywork. And extra appreciation also goes to Ian Kamm, of Sutherland-Chan School and Teaching Clinic, Toronto, Ontario, and Judy Dean, of Agua Dulce Center and Spa, Prescott, Arizona, for providing extensive review assistance and providing knowledgeable and insightful criticism for the benefit of future massage therapists.

The following individuals served as reviewers or provided other assistance in creating *The Business of Massage*:

The 2001 AMTA Council of Schools Board:
   Peggy Smith, BMSI Institute, Overland Park, Kansas
   Ron Garvock, North Vancouver, British Columbia
   Barry Antoniow, Kiné-Concept Institute Maritimes, Fredericton, New Brunswick
   Winona Bontrager, Lancaster School of Massage, Lancaster, Pennsylvania

Steve Albertson, Chicago School of Massage, Chicago, Illinois

Christopher Alvarado, Chicago School of Massage, Chicago, Illinois

John Balletto, Center for Muscular Therapy, Inc., and AMTA Foundation president, Providence, Rhode Island

James E. Barr, Jr., CPA, Barr &Associates, Overland Park, Kansas

Patricia Benjamin, Chicago School of Massage, Chicago, Illinois

Sue Brown, Illinois School of Health Careers, Chicago, Illinois

Kristin Chou, *etopa*, and the International Spa Association (ISPA), Hammond, Louisiana

Leslie Ciaccio, Kishwaukee College, Malta, Illinois

Judy Dean, Agua Dulce Center and Spa, Prescott, Arizona

René Evers, Baltimore School of Massage, Baltimore, Maryland

Réal Gaboriault, Kiné-Concept Institute, Montreal, Quebec

Claude Gagnon, Lakeside School of Massage Therapy, Milwaukee, Wisconsin

Ian Kamm, Sutherland-Chan School & Teaching Clinic, Toronto, Ontario

Carole Ostendorf, COMTA executive director, Evanston, Illinois

Jerry Pearce, Desert Institute of the Healing Arts, Tucson, Arizona

Sarah Rehwalt, COMTA commissioner, Portland, Oregon

Rhonda Reich, Boulder School of Massage, Boulder, Colorado

Demara Stamler, Potomac Massage Training Institute, Washington, DC

Diana Thompson, Hands Heal, Seattle, Washington

Diane Trieste, International Spa Association (ISPA), and COMTA commissioner, Canyon Ranch, Arizona

Jean Wible, Baltimore School of Massage, Baltimore, Maryland

TAKING STOCK of Your CAREER OPTIONS

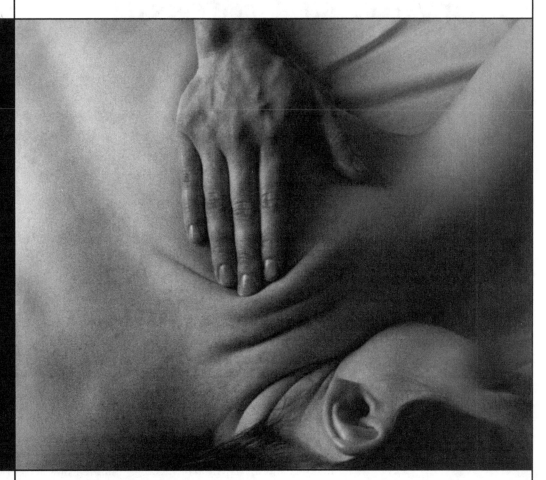

IN THIS CHAPTER, YOU'LL LOOK AT TWO PIECES OF THE PUZZLE:

1. Your career options as a massage therapist
2. Yourself

PUT THE TWO TOGETHER AND WHAT DO YOU SEE?

Chapter Objectives

1. Identify the scope and individual suitability of career opportunities available to massage therapists.

2. Identify self-assessment strategies for examining how your needs, behaviors, beliefs, and attitudes are relevant to the practice of massage therapy.

3. Identify how personal and cultural values, attitudes, and ethics influence the profession of massage therapy.

4. Identify the pros and cons of working in specific business structures.

Few fields of practice offer the variety or flexibility of options you'll find in massage therapy and bodywork. Before you start to explore these options, get your bearings by looking at the big picture. How did the practice of massage begin? How did it evolve? Where does it stand now, and —most importantly—where and how do you want to take your place in it?

Overview of Profession

You are entering a profession with a legacy rich in compassion, dedication to health and well-being, and high standards of practice. Almost every individual who chooses to become trained in massage does so because of a sincere desire to help people.

Shared Wisdom

"Attitude and determination are so important. Study to gather all the knowledge you can from what is presented to you. Don't just study enough to pass tests. The real test is when you apply service to the clients, so store all the information you can to insure safe, therapeutic, and professional services."

—Carrie Badker, "Carrie's Kadesh" School of Massage, Mitchell, South Dakota

As you complete your studies in anatomy, physiology, hands-on techniques, ethics, and other subjects, there's a good chance that you hold an image of yourself someday providing massage to benefit many people. You might have a particular type of client in mind—clients who appreciate the cumulative wellness effects of massage, women and men who seek relaxation and rejuvenation at spas, or athletes seeking relief from pain and injury.

Massage provides such rich benefits for its recipients— as more and more scientific research is validating—that it's unfortunate when excellent practitioners don't make a living at it. The Small Business Administration reports that just under 40 percent of small businesses that opened between 1989 and 1992 were still open six years later. Practitioners who care enough about staying in the profession must take seriously the work required to operate a profitable business.

Realism Comes Before Success

Many massage therapists are extremely good at running a business and supporting themselves financially, which enables them to practice the profession they love. But, if SBA statistics hold true for massage therapy practices, for every 10 massage therapists who are successful in their practices or careers, there are probably six who aren't. What a waste of gifts and skills, for someone to become trained as a massage therapist who could provide so much to so many, but who for lack of know-how is not able to make a living at it.

Some massage therapists support themselves within a year of opening a private practice. Those are the therapists who either have solid business and marketing experience under their belts, or are just plain lucky. They are not the majority. The majority take three or four years to establish a thriving business, and most of them work as employed massage therapists before they open their own practices.

Surviving Apprenticeship

When successful practitioners were asked to offer advice to new massage therapists and bodyworkers entering he profession, many of them said, "Spend at least your first three years working for someone else before you consider opening your own practice." One long-time practitioner put it in terms of having to "survive the apprenticeship" before you can fully and confidently find yourself an integrated member of this thriving and satisfying profession.

The most frequently cited reasons for advising new massage therapists to work as employees before opening their own practices were:

- To gain extensive hands-on practice to refine their technique— to establish confident touch and a comfortable rhythm and sequence of performing massages.
- To build stamina by working on as many as five to seven clients a day, an experience most students do not acquire in school practice clinics
- To gain skill-building relationships with a diversity of clients. Nowhere else will a practitioner gain such broad exposure to working with the public as he or she will as an employed massage therapist for a fitness center, clinic (i.e., massage, chiropractic, medical), or spa.

Many practitioners emphasized the need for enduring the rigors of apprenticeship in order to emerge as a fully functioning—in all facets of body, mind and spirit— massage therapist or bodyworker. They emphasized the reality of the start-up phase in order to give moral support to their new colleagues because of how deeply rewarding the profession becomes once someone becomes fully integrated into it and financially successful.

But before we go too far down the path of describing the pros and cons of various career or business opportunities, let's take a step back and look at where this profession started so you will know better how to find your place in it.

Ancient and Diverse History

The recorded history of massage goes back at least 4,000 years. Written and pictorial records from the ancient civilizations of Sumer, Egypt, China, India, Greece, and Rome contain descriptions of massage and exercises. Forms of massage developed originally in ancient China and India continue to this day in more modern forms of Asian bodywork, and the heritage of Greece and Rome is found in today's Western massage.

The development of massage therapy in modern Western culture can be traced to the 19th century, and the work of Per Henrik Ling of Sweden and Johann Georg Metzger of Amsterdam. The combined systems of Ling and Metzger, Swedish movements and massage, form the basis of today's Western massage.

In the first half of 20th century America, massage could be found at spas and hot springs, Turkish baths, natural healing resorts, health clubs, beauty salons, and Swedish massage establishments. The Greek and Roman tradition of massage for athletes was continued by athletic massage practitioners and trainers.

During the 1950s the practice of massage in the United States went into a period of decline. "Massage parlor" and "masseuse" changed from neutral descriptions to terms associated with prostitution and damaged the image of legitimate massage practitioners. Advances in conventional medicine overshadowed natural healing methods respected well in previous times, including massage.

Shared Wisdom

"To succeed in business you must first succeed in your own life. The successful massage business owners I know present a cheerful countenance and infectious enthusiasm, and are grounded in the belief in the value of what they are doing. They have resolved their personal issues to the point that their daily presentation lacks signs of anger and hostility. Their personal lives are stable. They are wholesome, outgoing people lovers. Doing the personal work early creates the situations that lead to a successful business."

—Ed Denning, Stark State College of Technology, Canton, Ohio

Shared Wisdom

"Be patient during the first year in practice. The first year is a good time to focus on technique and skill proficiency, as well as to develop a personal niche. Time spent in a supported environment, such as a chiropractic or multi-professional office, allows for development in these areas without the additional pressure of business development, marketing and advertising. It also allows time to build a client base and the funding necessary for private practice and increased business expenses."

—Ann Marie Engstrom, Rising Spirit Institute of Natural Health, Atlanta, Georgia

During the 1960-'70s, there was a revival of interest in massage in the United States. The Human Potential Movement and counterculture of that time produced a simplified and popular form of Swedish massage called Esalen Massage. In addition, health practices from other cultures, including China, Japan, and India, that included forms of massage were introduced to the general public. Athletes rediscovered sports massage as a way to improve performance, as well as help prevent and speed recovery from injuries. People began seeking more natural, holistic, and wellness-oriented approaches to health.

The growing interest in massage on a number of fronts in the 1970s fueled the revival of an economy related to massage. Fundamental to this economy is the increasing demand by the general public for massage, and the viability of massage therapy as a rewarding career. In the beginning of the 21st century, massage and bodywork are again part of mainstream health practices. Massage practitioners are recognized as better educated, more professional, and better skilled than ever before. [History overview abstracted from Tappan, F.M. and P.J. Benjamin. *Tappan's Handbook of Healing Massage Techniques: Classic, Holistic and Emerging Methods*. Stamford, CT: Appleton and Lange, 1998].

As you explore the wide variety of career options in massage therapy, you might want to give a nod of gratitude toward those who paved the way. Their legacy is your future in a rewarding career.

Know Yourself

Experience has shown that people are more likely to achieve their goals if they are clear about what they want. If you have known your entire life that you want to practice sports massage in the clinical setting of athletic sports medicine, you're home free once you have the proper training. You know what your goals are. But if you're like most people, you feel a definite attraction to some things and not others, but you haven't yet figured out what it all adds up to in terms of choosing a career direction.

Your beliefs, attitudes, and values have already influenced you in pursuing training in massage. They are derived from many sources of influence—the region where you grew up and live now, your family's traditions and beliefs about religion or spirituality, your socioeconomic background, your ethnic heritage, and your educational and work experience. See chapter 5 for more information about how your beliefs, attitudes, and values affect your practice.

Many tools are available to help you clarify how your interests and attractions can direct you to your career goals.

Self-Assessment Tools

Personality Tests and Interest Inventories

There are many tests and questionnaires that can help you better understand your interests and natural skills. The benefit of all of them is that they cause you to think about things you like and things you don't like, and in doing so to examine how your likes and dislikes fit into a career choice.

One of the best-known personality type indicators, the Myers-Briggs Type Indicator®, must be completed under the guidance of a qualified administrator, and is published by the Consulting Psychologists Press. Using the Myers-Briggs indicator, you learn valuable information about yourself in the following areas:

Introvert/Extrovert
Where, primarily, do you direct your energy? Is it to the outer world, through spoken words and action? Then, you are an extrovert. Or do you direct your energy to the inner world of thoughts and emotions?— an introvert.

Sensing/Intuitive
How do you prefer to process information? Do you prefer facts and figures and objective reality? If so, you are using "sensing" to process information. If you prefer to rely more on gut feel, and what might be rather than what is the current status, you would fall into the "intuitive" classification.

Thinking/Feeling
How do you prefer to make decisions? Similar to the distinctions between sensing and intuitive, the "thinking" personality type relies on logic, scientific analysis, and objective observation in making decisions. The "feeling" type depends more on subjective inputs, and tends to integrate qualities, such as appreciation and sympathy, into the equation before making a decision.

Judgment/Perception
How do you prefer to organize your life? If you are structured in your life organization—that is, you have a plan, you know where you stand in that plan, and you have contingencies built into your plan that address all the what-ifs life might throw at you—you're in the "judgment" classification. If, on the other hand, you discover life as you go along, and you like to keep your options open rather than make hard-and-fast decisions, you fall into the category of "perception."

Knowing where you fall in any of these classifications gives you information about yourself that is neither good nor bad. Knowing your personality indicators can help you a great deal in understanding how to work effectively with others, and in what type of practice environment you will be most comfortable.

Other personality and interest inventories include the Keirsey Temperament Sorter and the Enneagram. There are Web-based versions of personality and interest questionnaires, but be sure to respect the copyrights of these tools and take them only as directed. Some of these tests are available in abbreviated form for individuals to take if the tests are not being sold for commercial use.

Talk with Others, Get a Mentor

Don't limit yourself to just studying and practicing massage skills and reading about career options. Get specifics by building professional relationships. Talk to practicing therapists to learn what they experience in their work situations. In addition, find at least one mentor, a more experienced massage therapist who is willing to share his or her wisdom with you in an ongoing professional relationship. A mentor doesn't necessarily have to be another massage therapist. He or she might work in a related field and is familiar with the organization with which you want to work or with being an independent contractor or owner of a business.

Meet with your mentor regularly to talk and listen. As in any career, you are bound to have your ups and downs; a wise mentor can help you navigate them successfully. A successful career is a continual learning process.

Self-Evaluation: What Makes You Tick?

Take some time to reflect on how you would describe the career you want. Compare your image of yourself as a massage therapist with the actual opportunities in the field, which are described in the next section of this chapter. The time you spend reading, talking with others, and reflecting on insights about yourself, will help you plan a career that meets your professional, personal, and financial goals. As you answer the questions in the self-evaluation worksheet, "What Makes You Tick" (figure 1.1 page 7), remember that you are most likely to achieve personal, professional, and financial success if your career goals are compatible with your personal abilities, interests, character, and values.

If you are not sure about your strengths, ask people who know you well what they think your strengths are. It is important to be as honest as you can in self-evaluation, so you choose a career path that is realistic and satisfying.

After you have completed the worksheet, look over your answers. Can you begin to see the kind of work setting that would suit you best? For example, if you want to devote yourself to a particular kind of massage and minimize administrative activities, probably you would be happier as an employee than as an individual owner. If you are self-motivated and comfortable with risk, you would more likely enjoy being self-employed. But by being self-employed, you can plan on spending five to ten hours a week on recordkeeping, and another five hours a week on marketing. Your self-knowledge is the key to determining which career path is best for you. As an emerging profession, massage therapy offers tremendous opportunities.

Resources

Where to Find a Mentor
- at chapter or national meetings of your professional association
- through a massage therapist national directory
- at your school—look for teachers who show wisdom and an interest in students
- at a place of business you frequent or work
- among your colleagues—ask them to identify someone they particularly respect

---

Figure 1.1

You are most likely to achieve personal, professional, and financial success if your career goals are compatible with your personal abilities, interests, character, and values. It is important to be as honest as you can in the self-evaluation, to enable you to choose a career path that will be realistic and personally satisfying.

1. Why do you work? _____
   _____
   _____

2. What's important to you? (peace and quiet? intellectual stimulation? helping others? job security? expressing yourself creatively? spending time with your family? being independent?) _____
   _____
   _____

3. What types of activities give you satisfaction? (reading? balancing your checkbook? organizing an event? talking with a close friend? going to parties?) _____
   _____
   _____

4. What strengths (physical, mental, character, spiritual) do you have that can help you as a massage therapist?
   _____
   _____
   _____

5. What are your goals as an individual? _____
   _____
   _____

6. If you're part of a couple, what are your goals together? _____
   _____
   _____

7. What are your ambitions? _____
   _____
   _____

8. Describe the jobs you've enjoyed the most (before you became a massage therapist). _____
   _____
   _____

the
BUSINESS
of **MASSAGE**

© 2002 American Massage Therapy Association, Evanston, IL. *The Business of Massage*. All Rights Reserved. #20026

9. Describe the jobs you've enjoyed the least (before you became a massage therapist). _____

_____

_____

10. Do you prefer to work around other people or alone? _____

_____

11. Are you comfortable reporting to someone? If so, does it matter whether the person is a massage therapist or a non-massage-therapist manager? _____

_____

_____

12. What workplace values are essential to you? _____

_____

_____

13. Do you like to structure your own use of time, or do you prefer to let someone else set priorities and arrange schedules? _____

_____

14. Would you enjoy setting up the physical environment in which to provide massage, or would you prefer having this handled by someone else? _____

_____

15. Will massage therapy be your main or only source of income? (right away? in time?) _____

_____

_____

16. With what kinds of clients would you enjoy working? (babies? children? athletes? people with illnesses or special needs such as trauma or abuse victims? animals?) _____

_____

_____

17. Do you like telling people about the benefits of massage and encouraging them to try it?_____

_____

18. Do you enjoy paperwork? Avoid it?_____

_____

© 2002 American Massage Therapy Association, Evanston, IL. *The Business of Massage*. All Rights Reserved. 20026

19. Do you like performing a variety of business tasks each day and each week, or would you prefer to focus only on massage itself? _____

20. How many hours do you want to work each week? _____

21. How many of your work hours do you want to spend providing massages? (Consider your physical limitations as well as your financial goals.) _____

22. How many hours per week do you want to spend on paperwork, phone calls and marketing?_____

23. Do you like working the same hours each week, or do you prefer variety and/or flexibility? _____

24. What modalities of massage are you trained to offer? _____

25. Do you enjoy speaking before a group? _____

26. What additional skills, techniques, and/or modalities do you want to learn?_____

27. How many hours of continuing education per year do you plan to take? _____

28. Do you enjoy the theories behind massage therapy? _____

29. Would you enjoy researching or teaching?_____

30. Who has given you career guidance already or might be a mentor for you? _____

31. Do your family and friends support your career goals?_____

the
BUSINESS
of MASSAGE

© 2002 American Massage Therapy Association, Evanston, IL. *The Business of Massage*. All Rights Reserved. 20026

Know the Opportunities in the Field

Within the past few years, there has been a virtual explosion in the number of massage therapy and bodywork practitioners. Data from a 1998 study indicate that U.S. consumers are spending $4 to $6 billion each year on visits to massage therapists [Eisenberg, David, et al. "Trends in Alternative Medicine Use in the United States, 1990-1997." *Journal of the American Medical Association* 280(18), November 11, 1998, pages 1569-1575]. As more people appreciate the benefits of massage, massage therapists should be able to offer their professional services in a growing number of situations, to an ever-widening variety of clients.

Recent American Massage Therapy Association® (AMTA®) surveys indicate that members are seeking to increase the amount of time they practice in the area of prevention and wellness, and decrease the amount of time they work with clients for relaxation and stress management [source: American Massage Therapy Association Segmentation Study 2000]. This indicator probably does not mean that massage therapists are downplaying the importance of relaxation and stress management, but rather that they are broadening their professional viewpoints to the bigger picture of prevention and wellness, of which stress management is a subset.

People—potential massage clients—have many needs, and today they are looking for a way to satisfy these needs and to renew and enrich themselves. This is especially true of the baby boom generation, whose great size drives many trends in our society. Among the trends relevant to massage therapists are the following:

Need for Self-Direction to Enrich Quality of Life
People want to be able to call their own shots. Massage therapy allows people to do something about their health and well-being.

Need for Connection
As social beings, we want to be connected to others, but the time commitment one can give is reduced as a result of the two-income household, particularly in the United States. You should therefore consider how to make your service available to people when they need it.

Need for Everyday Celebration
People want to pamper themselves. You can position your service as a way people can pamper themselves and satisfy their need to celebrate.

Need for Inspiration
People are on a continual journey of self-improvement that leads to
realizing their potential and their ability to help others. Massage can
help people along this journey.

Adapted from "Living in a Kaleidoscope," presentation by Marty Horn, DDB Needham, at American
Marketing Association's *Cool Trends Hot Ideas: Maximizing Tomorrow's Marketing Opportunities,*
May 12, 1999.

See "Consumer Survey Facts" (figure 1.2, page 12) and "Who Becomes a
Massage Therapist" (figure 1.3, page 13) for trend data about growth in the
massage therapy profession.

Another trend in massage and bodywork is the increased funding of research into
the benefits of alternative therapies. The funding history of the National Center for
Complementary and Alternative Medicine of the National Institutes of Health
showed an increase from $2 million funded in 1992 to more than $68 million in
2000. This increased interest in alternative therapies has implications for massage
therapists who want to become more involved in research. It raises public awareness of the benefits of massage. Along with these trends, the use of complementary
medicine, including massage, is on the rise, as are wellness programs. As public
awareness rises, more people will seek massage for the first time, and you will have
the opportunity to develop long-term therapeutic relationships with them.

All these reasons for rapid growth are good news for you as a new practitioner.
Your clients may be infants or adults, athletes, medical patients, or even animals.
Among the many options for a massage career are practices devoted exclusively
to massage in medical settings such as clinics and hospitals, and other facilities
such as cruise ships, resorts, and fitness centers.

"Full-time and Part-time Income of AMTA Members" (figure 1.4, page 14) and
"Average Fees Charged by Massage Therapists Nationwide" (figure 1.5 page 14)
provide a general idea of the income range you might earn as a massage therapist.
In 2001, AMTA estimated that fees ranged from $45 to $75 for a 60-minute session.

The variety of settings in which you can perform massage and bodywork is broad
enough to suit a wide range of career interests. In the following section, we look at
opportunities in the field for practitioners in these settings:

medical
spas
wellness
fitness/sports
specialty

Figure 1.2 Consumer Survey Facts

The following are findings of a survey conducted by the Opinion Research Corporation, Princeton, New Jersey, and commissioned by the American Massage Therapy Association. The survey was conducted July 26-29, 2001, among a national probability sample of 1,000 adults (501 men and 499 women) ages 18 and older, living in private households in the continental United States. This survey has been conducted annually since June 1997. It is used here with permission from the American Massage Therapy Association.

- More than twice as many adult Americans report receiving one or more massages from a massage therapist in the past year (17%) as did in 1997 (8%).

- In 2001, 27% of Americans said they had had a massage in the past five years, compared to 17% in 1997 who said they had had a massage in the previous five years.

- In 2001, 24% of Americans said they expect to get a massage in the next 12 months, compared to 21% in 2000 who expected to do so.

- Twenty-five percent of adults with family incomes of $50,000+ had a massage from a massage therapist in the past 12 months.

- Locations where clients received massage:
  Day spa: 17%   Medical clinic: 3%
  Massage therapist's office: 14%   Workplace: 3%
  Client's home: 10%   Student clinic: 2%
  Chiropractor's office: 9%   Hospital: 2%
  Beauty salon: 7%   Retail outlet: 1%
  Health club: 7%   Physician's office: 1%
  Hotel/resort: 5%   Miscellaneous locations: 13%

- Region and Massage
  West Coast: 22%
  North Central: 20%
  Northeast: 14%
  South: 13%

- More people in the West (29%) and Northeast (26%) expect to get a massage in the next 12 months.

For updated information when new surveys are conducted, visit the AMTA Web site at www.amtamassage.org®, and go to the Massage Information Center section.

Figure 1.3   Who Becomes a Massage Therapist?

A 2000 survey of member demographics conducted by the American Massage Therapy Association reflected the following information about who are massage therapists. It is used here with permission from the American Massage Therapy Association.

- Gender: More than three-quarters are female.
  80% female
  20% male

- Age: Two-thirds are between the ages of 35 and 54.
  25% are 21-34
  61% are 35-54
  14% are 55+
  Average age 42.6

- Areas of Work: Type of work is fairly evenly balanced.
  20% relaxation
  19% stress management
  17% prevention/wellness
  17% chronic pain management
  16% injury rehabilitation
  4.7% spirituality
  4.5% special luxury
  1.8% other

- Education: Compared to the national average, practitioners are highly educated.
  90% attended some college
  46% have earned at least a bachelor's degree
  10% no college

- Practice Time:
  Part-time: 59% (defined as fewer than 17 one-hour sessions per week)
  Full-time: 41% (more than 17 paid hours of massage per week, plus administrative duties of running their business)

- Income:
  Full-time: average $32,500/year
  Part-time: average $12,000/year
  Practitioners in large population areas tend to earn more than the average because of higher cost of living in those areas and greater number of potential clients.

Figure 1.4 Full-time and Part-time Income of AMTA Members

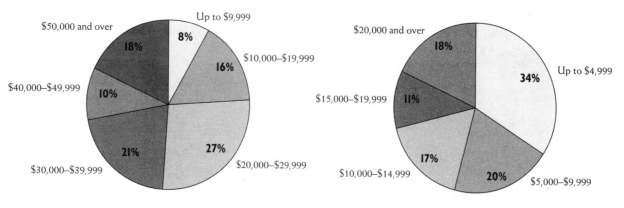

Full-time Massage Income

Part-time Massage Income

Note: Massage therapists who practice in areas with populations of at least 500,000 tend to earn higher incomes, reflecting the higher cost of living and the greater number of potential clients.

Figure 1.5 Average Fees Charged by Massage Therapists Nationwide

Geographic Regions

Length of Sessions	Total	New England	NY/NJ	Mid Atl	Midwest	Southeast	Southwest	Plains	High Plains	Northwest	West
15 Minute	$16	$13	$15	$15	$13	$27	$15	$16	$12	$15	$16
30 Minute	$20	$29	$32	$26	$26	$31	$27	$28	$24	$29	$30
45 Minute	$40	$41	$45	$42	$37	$46	$40	$43	$28	$39	$44
60 Minute	$40	$52	$55	$49	$43	$52	$47	$43	$40	$47	$50
90 Minute	$61	$70	$81	$70	$63	$75	$70	$65	$59	$65	$71
120 Minute	$91	$85	$108	$92	$84	$97	$90	$81	$85	$85	$97

New England - Vermont, New Hampshire, Massachusetts, Rhode Island, Connecticut
Mid-Atlantic - Pennsylvania, West Virginia, Maryland, Delaware, District of Columbia
Midwest - Minnesota, Wisconsin, Illinois, Indiana, Ohio, Michigan
Southeast - Kentucky, Tennessee, North Carolina, Georgia, Alabama, Mississippi, Florida
Southwest - Louisiana, Arkansas, Oklahoma, New Mexico
Plains - Nebraska, Iowa, Missouri, Kansas
High Plains - Montana, North Dakota, South Dakota, Wyoming, Utah, Colorado
Northwest - Washington, Oregon, Idaho
West - California, Nevada, Arizona

Source: American Massage Therapy Association, *1998 General Membership Survey: Final Executive Report.*

The Medical Market

As the practice of massage therapy grows in acceptance by both consumers and the medical community, opportunities for massage therapists grow. According to a survey conducted by the American Massage Therapy Association in 2000, roughly three-quarters of its members would like to work with medical doctors, although not necessarily on-site in a medical facility. Members also reported that more than half of them receive more referrals from the medical community than they did two years ago.

The results of a survey conducted in the state of Washington indicate strong recognition on the part of health clinicians that massage is effective. In Washington, where complementary and alternative medicine (CAM) providers have been recognized by health plans since 1996, the survey asked medical practitioners five years later, in 2000, what they thought of CAM practices. Of 12 CAM practices surveyed, massage therapy was ranked highest (74%) in terms of being perceived as always or usually effective. The next closest CAM practice in the same category of effectiveness was acupuncture, ranked by 67.7% of clinician respondents ["Post-Legislative Mandate: Two-Thirds of Group Health Clinician Respondents View CAM as Effective." *The Integrator for the Business of Alternative Medicine,* April 2001].

Another study showing the increased acceptance of CAM practices was published by the American Medical Association in September 2000, which said two-thirds of the nation's medical schools teach herbal therapy, acupuncture, massage, or other alternative medicine [source: Barzansky, et al. "Educational Programs in US Medical Schools, 1999-2000." *Journal of the American Medical Association* 284:1114-1120 September 6, 2000]. These results do not necessarily suggest that it is medical massage that is sought, but only that the medical community increasingly accepts massage as a complementary therapy.

Massage therapists' views about participation with insurance and healthcare reimbursement vary widely by region. Third party reimbursement is widely accepted in the West and in Florida, and less common in other areas of the country. Another trend indicated by the AMTA survey is that newer practitioners—those who have been in the field for less than four years—are more likely to participate in third-party reimbursement than are longer-experienced practitioners.

The range of possibilities for working with medical practitioners is growing, especially in the eastern states and the Midwest. Possibilities include such places and practices as the following:

addiction counseling centers—mostly volunteer	obstetric practice
athletic training	orthopedic physician practice
chiropractic practice	pediatric practice
hospices—mostly volunteer	physical therapy clinics
medical clinics	physician family practice
naturopathic practice	rehabilitation centers
nursing homes	rheumatology practice
	sports medicine clinics

Shared Wisdom

"Anyone who has been in the field of massage therapy and bodywork for more than five years has done a lot of personal growth work. Some types of practices place greater emphasis on the mind/spirit aspects of massage, and some on the physical aspects. When a person has a foot in both camps—when the session is nurturing, kind, and healing, as well as physically excellent—the more value it imparts to the client and to the world at large."

—Judy Dean, Agua Dulce Center and Spa, Prescott, Arizona

As health benefits of massage become more broadly accepted, there are more opportunities to collaborate with medical practitioners. You might expand your working relationship with the medical community in any of the following ways:

- hired as employee
- hired as contractor
- practice on-site by appointment
- accept referrals to your practice

Do your homework before you contact professionals who work in medical settings. Schools that provide specialty training in medical massage teach the following subjects to students who want to provide complementary massage within a medical setting:

Pathophysiology
This is the study of specific medical conditions. Massage therapists need to understand not only the appropriate massage and bodywork techniques for a particular condition but also the medical treatment. Knowledge of pathophysiology helps you determine cautions and contraindications for a variety of medical conditions, and to know when it is appropriate to refer a client to another specialist.

Medical Modalities
Learn about modalities used in medical settings, such as electrotherapy, ultrasound, electrical stimulation, and pharmacology. Learn your state's regulations that govern various modalities. For example, in some states, massage therapists are allowed to perform ultrasound tests. In others, they are not.

Techniques
Learn appropriate techniques for a variety of medical conditions and diseases. Neuromuscular work is most common. Some medical conditions, such as burns, require non-touch types of body therapy, such as energy modalities.

Communication Skills and Recordkeeping
Familiarity with medical terminology and recordkeeping specific to different types of medical practice is key to gaining credibility in these settings. Good communication also requires understanding organizational structures and chains of command typical in particular medical settings.

Source: Jean Wible and René Evers, Medical Massage Program, Baltimore School of Massage, Baltimore, Maryland.

Shared Wisdom

"I have found that the fastest way to establish credibility with the medical community is to have them see that you are not just someone seeking referrals, but a fellow health-care practitioner who can make a difference to his or her patients. They are used to empirical evidence and double-blind studies that prove efficaciousness."

—Bob Haase,
Bodymechanics School of Myotherapy & Massage, Olympia, Washington

According to an AMTA member survey taken in 2000, many practitioners who work in medical settings view the practice of massage and bodywork as a medical modality rather than as a personal care service. To them, the practice is legitimized due to its collaboration with allopathic medicine. It is not unusual for a nurse or physical therapist to train in massage therapy, or for a massage therapist to become trained in nursing, and to find a satisfying career mix in combining the two professions. The AMTA survey also indicated that members who work in medical settings showed the highest incomes for massage therapy, and that they work the most hours.

Another avenue for combining massage and medical practices is to work as an independent contractor at a medical establishment, or to accept and make referrals. Of the massage therapists who work with the medical profession, about three-quarters of them work with chiropractors, and more than half work with medical doctors.

The Spa Market

The spa industry is one of the fastest growing segments of career opportunities for massage therapists. An estimated 5,689 spas throughout the United States employ approximately 151,000 people, two-thirds of whom are full-time. The number of spas has doubled in the past five years, and the number of employees doubled between 1997 and 1999. In 1999, there were more than 88.6 million spa visits made in the United States. Of the nearly $38 billion leisure market, spa services make up approximately $5 billion [The International Spa Association's *2000 Spa Industry Study*, conducted and prepared by PriceWaterhouseCoopers, January 2001].

The spa industry has grown from an exclusive luxury of which wealthy, pampered women availed themselves, to one that embraces people of all levels of income, age, and gender, who are interested in body, mind, and spirit balance.

Many massage therapists view spas as a good way to get experience when they first start their careers. A practitioner can gain invaluable experience working in an efficient business setting and learning good skills at communicating effectively with a broad variety of clients. But don't make the mistake of assuming that spas are only for entry level careers. The best spas have excellent employee longevity.

There are essentially four types of spas:

Destination Spa
This means that the spa is "the whole event"—it is all-inclusive, and guests usually select one of several packages of services for an entire week or partial week.

Day Spa
Day spas make up about three-quarters of the spa industry. This is where you'll find a salon of spa services, and you go by appointment. This could even be at a fitness center. You do not stay overnight.

Shared Wisdom

"If you worked in a spa for even one year, you would triple your experience in hands-on/technical skills and strengthen your ability to relate to new clients, relative to any other work experience. Spas offer very eclectic experiences which relate to health and wellness."

—*Di Trieste, Corporate Spa Treatment Director, Canyon Ranch Health Resorts, Tucson, Arizona*

Resort Spa

The spa is located within a hotel or complex; the spa is almost always independently owned and managed. It can have a focus on a specialty, such as fitness, burnout, rejuvenation, or beauty.

Cruise Ships

Most cruise ships have spas, which are basically like resort spas except they are on cruise ships.

The watchword in spas is productivity. The well-managed spa is designed to serve its clients in a manner that is both relaxing and efficient. Efficiency on the part of spa staff is necessary because of the need to seamlessly schedule multiple clients to take the most advantage of spa services and to improve profitability of the business.

Key Trends in the Spa Industry

PRODUCTS: Spas are focusing on a more holistic approach. While the traditional esthetician services continue to be offered, spas are expanding their Asian-modality treatments and fitness components.

CONSUMER: Consumers view spas as a place where they can escape from the stresses of daily life. A focus on health puts a greater emphasis on prevention and fitness.

INVESTMENTS: Spas are a main component of any new resort being built or renovated. Malls are adding day spas. Competition is expected to come increasingly from the cosmetic industry and traditional hair salons. The medical community is also investing in the spa industry.

TECHNOLOGY: The spa industry uses the Internet in their advertising and in understanding customers. But the industry's focus is "touch," not "technology" oriented.

Source: The International SPA Association's *2000 Spa Industry Study,* conducted and prepared by PriceWaterhouseCoopers, January 2001.

If you are interested in developing your practice in the spa industry, seek training in content and skills that will make you an asset to the spa business before you apply for a job at one. The Commission on Massage Therapy Accreditation (COMTA) recommends that a well-rounded educational program for prospective spa employees include information in the following areas:

- History, philosophy, and culture of the spa experiences

- Introduction to various types of spa environments

- Physiological effects of thermals, including but not limited to products, baths, and aromatherapy

- Indications, contraindications, and considerations of various spa modalities or approaches

- Sanitation as it relates to equipment, tools, and products

- Structure and function of the human body as it specifically relates to the spa services and to biochemical changes within the body as a result of spa modalities

- Self-care for practitioner, including but not limited to body mechanics, time management, and organization

- Introduction to modalities: overview of spa modalities

- Communication as it relates to guest services and education within the spa environment

- Safety as it relates to working in a spa environment

If you desire to work in the spa industry but your school does not provide this type of training, you might check out opportunities to take continuing education at regional conferences or other schools of massage therapy.

Probably the biggest learning curve a massage therapist will benefit from when he or she accepts a job at a spa will stem from the fact that he or she will be expected to do more than just give massages. Most spas are not geared to staffing employees who perform only one specialty service; they must rely on their employees to perform a broad range of functions. These functions might include providing guest services such as reception duties and folding towels. Performing a variety of functions helps to reduce burn-out, as you are expanding your skills in actually running a business, while you get necessary breaks from performing end-to-end massages.

The important thing to remember at a spa is that you are essentially working in a corporate environment. This means that your options for career growth are almost unlimited in terms of branching out in many directions within the health and wellness environment. In a well-run spa, you need to be an enthusiastic team player whose energy is directed to helping the spa serve its guests in the best way possible, both from a guest satisfaction and a profitability standpoint.

Spas are an excellent place to start a massage therapy career, for two reasons. One, they give the new practitioner an opportunity to build stamina and improve techniques from the experience of working on numerous clients. And two, spas expose the new practitioner to a wide diversity of clients, allowing him or her to refine his or her personal interaction and customer service skills.

Resources

Information about Spa Careers
- Capellini, Steve. *Massage Therapy Career Guide for Hands-On Success.* Milady Salon Ovations, 1999.
- International SPA Association (ISPA), 2365 Harrodsburg Rd., Suite A325, Lexington, KY 40504; Tel. (859) 226-4372; www.experienceispa.com
- Spa Jobs: www.spajobs.com
- Spa Massage Alliance, 1636 W. 1st Avenue, Spokane, WA 99204-0620; www.spamassagealliance.com

---

The Wellness Market

Wellness programs emphasize promoting and maintaining health rather than on treating illness or disease. They are based on models that focus attention on mind, body, and spirit, and to the total environment in which a person lives. The emphasis on wellness rather than on disease has been shown to reduce employee absenteeism, reduce the number of sick days and hours lost from work, and reduce overall healthcare costs. See chapter 5 for more information on the wellness model.

Companies and health centers that recognize the value of promoting wellness provide an appropriate and welcoming work setting for massage therapists and bodyworkers.

A study described in the National Wellness Association's newsletter [Chapman, Larry S. "Update on the Cost-Effectiveness of Worksite Health Promotion Programs" *Wellness Management*, Winter 1997, Vol. 13, No. 4] reported the following benefits at more than thirty companies that had studied the effects of wellness programs over a 15-year period:

- average days of sick leave reduced by 22%
- number of hospital admissions reduced by 62%
- number of physician visits reduced by 16%
- per capita health costs reduced by 28%
- injury incidence reduced by 25%
- per capita workers' compensation cost reduced by 47%

Because of the extensive benefits wellness programs offer, these programs can be found in many environments and are available to many segments of the population. In your own community, you might find wellness centers at any of the following locations:

colleges and universities   medical clinics
community-based wellness centers   retirement communities
company work sites   substance abuse centers
state and local government offices   women's health centers
hospitals

One attribute common to all wellness settings is focus on the health of the entire person. It is always important that a massage therapist is a role model in self-care, and it is especially important in wellness settings. Clients will be alert to a wellness practitioner's eating habits, mental and emotional well-being, and physical health and vitality. See chapter 6 for more information on self-care and its importance to clients.

Wellness settings provide great opportunities for client education. Clients are likely to be interested in knowing how massage and related holistic health practices affect their health. Working in a wellness setting can provide opportunities to partner with other health professionals, such as nutrition specialists, yoga and other fitness or spiritual practitioners, and meditation leaders, to provide your clients with a well-rounded menu of wellness practices.

Components of Wellness Programs

Wellness programs can include any of these components:

breast examination	diversity training	fitness training and classes
healing gardens	health club classes	health evaluation
job counseling	massage and bodywork	nap rooms
nutrition counseling	mental health counseling	smoking cessation
stress reduction training	tai chi	weight loss clinics
workplace safety	yoga	

The Fitness/Sports Market

The last several decades have witnessed a dramatic rise in the level of athletic performance. This increase can be attributed to improved technology and equipment, enhanced understanding of how nutrition fuels the body, enlightenment about psychological aspects of competition, and scientific advances in the study of body structure and function. The growing awareness of sports massage as a valuable addition to other physical therapies has become a key component in athletes' training regimens.

Some of the benefits of sports massage to the athlete or fitness enthusiast are:
- reduced chance of injury, both through education about preparation, as well as through deep tissue massage
- improved range of motion, strength, performance times
- shortened recovery time between workouts
- maximized supply of nutrition and oxygen through increased blood flow

Careers in fitness/sports massage can be found in many of the following settings:
- college and university sports teams
- professional sports teams
- sports massage clinics
- health and fitness centers
- rehabilitation clinics
- athletic resorts
- golf resorts and clubs

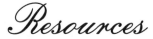

Resources

Information About Wellness Programs
Visit the sites below to learn more about wellness and to find out where national and regional conferences are held.

- Association for Worksite Health Promotion: www.awhp.org
- FitWell Associates, Inc.: www.fitwellinc.com/impact.html
- Health Enhancement Research Organization: www.the-hero.org
- HealthWorld Online: www.healthy.net
- National Wellness Institute: www.nationalwellness.org
- Wellness Councils of America: www.welcoa.org
- Wellness Web: www.wellweb.com

Sports massage practice can be categorized as maintenance or as event-related. Maintenance is integrated into a client's training program. It is regularly scheduled and proactive. A sports massage practitioner needs to have a thorough understanding of anatomy and kinesiology, along with expert knowledge of which muscles are used in a given sport and which are likely candidates for trouble. Zeroing in on particular muscle systems and working specific tissues go a long way toward building optimal conditioning and preventing strain and injury. The objective of a maintenance program is to help the athlete reach optimal performance through injury-free training.

Sports massage is used pre-event, when it supplements an athlete's warm-up to enhance circulation and reduce excess muscle and mental tension prior to competition. It improves tissue pliability and assists in metabolic exchange, readying the athlete for top performance. It is also used post-event, when it is geared toward reducing the trauma that occurs after the cessation of vigorous exercise. Helped by massage, the body is able to gradually slow down yet maintain oxygen flow to tired muscles still requiring elevated levels of oxygen.

The Specialty Markets

In addition to the varied mainstream environments in which to practice massage therapy, several specialties have emerged that broaden your options further. These specialties may be practiced as sole pursuits, or in conjunction with a mainstream practice. Specific training is available in all of these areas, and many of them offer certification that indicates your advanced training.

Animal Massage

Sometimes massage therapists develop animal massage as a specialty area, and sometimes veterinarians or veterinary technicians become certified in animal massage specialties so they can integrate these skills into their regular vet practices. The most common animal specialties are in canine and equine (horse) massage.

The International Association of Equine Sports Massage Therapists has approved a curriculum for this type of specialty, which results in a certificate in Equine Sports Massage Therapy. Benefits of equine massage are particularly helpful to performance horses that need to be in top form to compete. Equine massage also helps horses heal faster from muscle injuries than if they hadn't received massage. Practitioners trained in equine massage might work for owners and trainers in the horse racing world as well as the show arena.

In equine massage, you might find need for massage services at boarding stables, racetracks, and with law enforcement agencies that use horses in their line of work. If you practice canine massage, some of the options available to you are in working at dog agility trials, dog shows, dog flyball, doggie day care, and at vets' offices.

Shared Wisdom

"If you want to develop a specialty in canine massage, spend as much time as you can learning dog behavior, visit with veterinarians, go to dog shows and doggie day care, and take a certification program whose teachings include anatomy, pathology, and lots of hands-on massage."

—*Rhonda Reich, Boulder College of Massage*

The benefits of massage to animals are similar to the benefits to humans:
- maintaining muscle tone and flexibility
- increased blood and lymph circulation
- relieving discomfort from arthritis, lameness and hip dysplasia
- preventing injuries
- recovery from skeletal and muscular surgery or injury
- preventative overall health care
- relieving muscle pain by releasing endorphins

Source: Boulder College of Massage Therapy canine massage certification program.

Pregnancy and Infant Massage

Women can benefit from massage while they are pregnant, during labor, and after the birth. Pregnancy has a significant impact, not only on the mother's habits and lifestyle, but on her body, too, as it alters to accommodate the new life within it. Finding ways to manage extra stress during this time is essential at every stage of pregnancy, from conception to birth, and afterward during the postpartum period. Massage has also been shown to be beneficial to infants.

Benefits Before the Birth
- stress reduction
- increased flow of oxygen and blood to tissues, accelerating nutrients to mother and baby
- relief of backaches and other pains often experienced with pregnancy
- decreased swelling and edema as it can drain toxins from the mother's body
- help in coming to terms with evolving body image

Benefits During Labor
- reduce discomfort of repeatedly tensing muscles
- revitalize by relaxing the mother between contractions
- a partner or spouse can learn simple techniques to aid labor in this way

Benefits after the Birth
- speeds recovery from stress

Benefits of Massaging Baby
- helps infant digest feedings better
- helps build muscle tone, coordination and brain functioning
- stimulates circulation, helping to heal any birth-related trauma
- calms the baby's nervous system
- establishes a pattern of relaxation at an early age
- counterbalances frightening, negative messages about touch
- helps the mother or partner and the baby grow closer to each other

The International Association of Infant Massage (IAIM) was founded in the early 1980s. Its mission is "to promote nurturing touch and communication through training, education, and research so that parents, caregivers, and children are loved, valued, and respected throughout the world community."

Therapists who want to be certified as Certified Pregnancy Massage Therapists may do so through the National Association of Pregnancy Massage Therapy (NAPMT). NAPMT states that the goal of Certified Pregnancy Massage Therapists is "to provide therapeutic bodywork which focuses on the special needs of the mother-to-be as her body goes through the dramatic changes of the child-birth experience—pregnancy, birth, and post-partum."

Massage for Elderly

People over 75 constitute the fastest growing segment of the U.S. population. By 2020, one in five Americans will be over 60, according to the Population Reference Bureau, a nonprofit demographic study group. In "Massage for Elders: An Ever-Growing Opportunity" [*Massage Therapy Journal*, Fall 2001], Joan Lohman, a certified massage therapist who operates a successful practice serving "the age group society treats as 'the untouchables,'" provides an overview of her practice.

Benefits of Massage for Elders

- reduces stress
- deepens relaxation
- deepens breathing
- lowers blood pressure
- stimulates circulation
- relieves joint pain
- reduces swelling and edema

- stimulates bowels
- stimulates flow of lymph
- improves sleep
- releases endorphins
- decreases fear and anxiety
- brings sense of well-being
- decreases isolation

Practical Tips

- Have a client write his or her check before she/he comes to the session.
- Encourage your client to dress simply.
- Support the client to do as much dressing and undressing for herself/himself as she/he is able and time allows.
- Ask your client if she/he prefers to be nude or partially clothed.
- Allow extra time for small buttons and support hose, if client uses them.

Communication Pointers

- Call elders the night before or day of an appointment as a courtesy reminder.
- To avoid early wake-up calls, use a phone machine or telephone answering service. Elders are often up early, and may assume that the rest of the world arises by that hour.
- Speak clearly and strongly to the hearing-impaired.

- Let clients decide if they will keep hearing devices on during a massage.
- Avoid touching the ears when devices are on. It sets off a buzz.

Billing
- Many clients will write their own checks.
- In some cases, you may bill a family member or conservator.
- Some insurance companies will cover massage as a medical necessity.

Source: Joan S. Lohman. "Massage for Elders: An Ever-Growing Opportunity." *Massage Therapy Journal*, Fall 2001, pages 60-74.

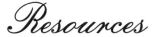

Information About Specialty Massage Careers
- Canadian Sport Massage Therapists Assn., P.O. Box 1330, Unity, Saskatchewan, S0K 4L0 Canada; (306) 228-2808; www.csmta.ca
- International Association of Equine Sports Massage Therapists, P.O. Box 447, Round Hill, VA 20141; www.iaesmt.com (includes canine specialty)
- International Association of Infant Massage (IAIM) - U.S. Chapter, 1891 Goodyear Avenue, Suite 622, Ventura, CA 93003; (805) 644-8524; www.iaim-us.com
- The National Association of Pregnancy Massage Therapy (NAPMT), 1007 MoPac Circle, Suite 202, Austin, TX 78746; 1-888-451-4945; www.napmt.home.texas.net
- U.S. Sports Massage Federation/International Sports Massage Federation, 2156 Newport Blvd., Costa Mesa, CA 92627; (949) 642-0735

Two Massage Careers

Jeanne Wagner's first career was as a registered nurse, but she soon longed to exchange high-tech care for a more high-touch career. She studied massage at the Lakeside School of Natural Therapeutics in Milwaukee, then worked part-time at a hospital, a group home for Alzheimer's patients, and several health centers. Those experiences helped Wagner refine her career goals, so she was ready when two hospitals wanted her to provide massages in their new in-house massage services. A year later, she had to hire people to keep up with the growing demand at the first two hospitals and to expand to two more.

Paul Jantzi always was interested in bodywork. He started with a small private practice and built his massage therapy career gradually as he gained networking skills. His first break came when he joined the La Mancha Athletic Club in Phoenix. From there, Jantzi went on to work in a variety of health club, resort, and clinical settings until professional contacts led him to a position at Valley Therapy Center, a busy Scottsdale, Arizona, clinic. He sees a combination of clients referred by doctors and private clients. He helps to provide relief for a variety of ailments, ranging from migraines to chronic fatigue syndrome. One reason he likes working at Valley Therapy is that he is part of a team.

Sources: Beata M. Hayton and Jeanne Wagner, R.N. "Do It in the Hospital," *Massage Therapy Journal* Spring 1999, pages 98-100, 102, 104; Mirka Knaster, and Paul Jantzi. "Offer Massage & Nutriceuticals", *Massage Therapy Journal,* Fall 1998, pages 100-107.

Know Who You Want to Work For

You know you want to practice massage. You might also have an idea of the type of client you would like to attract. Now add to your options the work environment you would most enjoy. Your basic choices are between being an employee and being self-employed. The choices in employment (full-time or part-time) and self-employment (independent contractor, sole proprietorship, partnership, or corporation) come in many varieties. There are pros and cons to each choice, and you are the only one who knows which one is better suited to you, at different points in your career.

Begin by envisioning the type of career you would like to have. Do you see yourself working alone or with others? Are you working in space you own or rent, or at someone else's facility, such as a health club or clinic? Who finds your clients and schedules your appointments?

The more you can answer questions such as these and create a mental picture of the kind of career you want, the better able you will be to make decisions about how you want to practice. For example, you can decide whether you want to work for yourself or for someone else. If you will be self-employed, you can decide whether to work alone or to create some type of organization.

Employee or Self-Employed?

For some people, a career in massage therapy is an opportunity to be out on their own. For others, this kind of liberty is not at all appealing. They prefer to work as employees of an organization in which others handle most of the paperwork, marketing, building maintenance, and other important support details.

Figure 1.6 Self-Employment Pros and Cons

PROS

- control over work standards
- control over hours
- authority to determine scope of services
- ability to reduce taxes by writing off expenses
- no upper limit on income if practice succeeds
- opportunity to be creative

CONS

- obligation to know and follow government regulations for businesses
- responsibility for finding and keeping clients
- responsibility for accounting and other administrative tasks
- responsibility for self-employment and Medicare taxes and benefits such as health and disability insurance, paid vacation time, and sick leave
- expenses of starting up and running a business
- risks of running a business, including financial risks (such as fluctuating income) and security risks (especially if working alone)
- potential for isolation and loneliness

Source: Sohnen-Moe, Cherie. "Practice Management, Part I." *Massage Therapy Journal*, Fall 1997, pages 141-142, 144.

Being Your Own Boss

Self-employment has some obvious attractions, some of which are listed in "Self-Employment Pros and Cons" (figure 1.6, page 29). For example, you can set your own work standards and hours. You decide where to work and the kinds of services you offer. You can emphasize the kinds of therapy and benefits that you consider the most worthwhile. The business you establish is your own practice.

Self-employment also can offer practical benefits. Your income potential is as unlimited as your potential to attract and meet the needs of clients. At the same time, you can use the expenses of operating your practice to reduce your taxable income. For example, if you buy office equipment you might be able to deduct the expense. If you make a house call, you might be able to write off a portion of the travel expense. And if you operate your practice out of your home, you can probably deduct a variety of business costs.

Self-employment also has a downside. Your income varies according to the number of clients you see and the number of days you work, and it is often hard to predict what you will earn from month to month. Also, you will have start-up expenses, so you might need another source of funds while you are waiting for your first payments from clients. If you start out smaller than anticipated, your income may be disappointing. Yet even if you provide massages only a few hours a month, you are legally considered a business, so you have all the responsibilities of any business owner.

You must follow the laws and regulations that apply where you are located. You must determine what taxes you owe, so you have to maintain careful records of your earnings and expenses. Additionally, self-employed people are responsible for paying the share of taxes that employers pay on behalf of their employees.

Running a practice involves other responsibilities as well. Finding and keeping clients can be a challenge. You must be sure that you or someone you trust is collecting your fees. If you maintain a space in which to practice, you must be sure it looks professional, feels comfortable, and meets building codes. Even if you hire people to handle some of these tasks, you, as the owner of the practice, are responsible for ensuring that the work is done properly. All this can be especially challenging when you are just starting out as a massage therapist.

Self-employment also has financial implications. Being able to write off expenses is nice, but you have to spend your own money first. Also, any benefits, such as time off and health insurance, will reduce your business's earnings.

Being an Employee

For some people, at certain stages of their career, the responsibilities of owning a practice are simply too overwhelming, or they just are not interested in owning a practice. They prefer working for someone else, especially because they can gain expertise early in their careers. Many therapists are able to arrange jobs that meet their personal needs for work hours, type of practice, and other criteria. They appreciate being in a situation in which someone else handles marketing, bookkeeping, and the many other responsibilities of running a business. They like getting a regular paycheck, with all the tax deductions properly made. They may also appreciate the opportunity to watch more experienced people and to learn the details of running a practice. These benefits are summarized in "Employment Pros and Cons" (figure 1.7, page 31).

Figure 1.7   Employment Pros and Cons

PROS

Employee:

*   learns from and possibly gets support from other employee practitioners in the company
*   learns his/her marketable attributes relative to co-worker practitioners
*   moves on without worrying about recovering an investment

Employer:

*   provides a steady paycheck
*   handles responsibilities of running a business, including paperwork and security
*   pays share of social security taxes and may provide benefits, such as paid vacation and health insurance

CONS

*   Employee must handle the organization's "office politics."
*   Employer pays practitioner only a portion of the client fee.
*   Employer determines business policies and working conditions.
*   Work hours may not be flexible.

Adapted from Sohnen-Moe, Cherie. "Practice Management, Part I." *Massage Therapy Journal*, Fall 1997, pages 141-142, 144.

Employee or Independent Contractor?

Some people try to get the best of both worlds by working at someone else's facility, such as a clinic or health club, not as employees but as independent contractors. Independent contractors have the benefit of writing off some of their expenses on their tax returns, but they let someone else run the facility at which they perform services.

If you want to be an independent contractor, understand that, for tax purposes, the IRS has guidelines for distinguishing an independent contractor from an employee. See "Employee or Independent Contractor" (figure 1.8, page 32).

The downside of being an employee is that you give up some control. If you work on Tuesday evenings, you may not be able to get that evening off to celebrate your child's birthday. If you would like to try expanding the types of services you offer, you probably will have to obtain permission first from your employer. If you think the facilities could use an upgrade, you will have to sell your ideas to someone else. And sometimes an employer over-schedules massage therapists, leaving them too little time between appointments for proper self-care.

Figure I.8 EMPLOYEE OR INDEPENDENT CONTRACTOR?

Check each of the following statements that describes your work.

❑ You decide how, when, and where you will perform your work.

❑ You know how to provide the services; the company that contracted with you did not train you in its procedures.

❑ Your services are not something the company has made part of its operations.

❑ You do not personally provide some of the massages or other services for which you are paid. (For example, you hire an assistant to do some of the work.)

❑ Any assistants you use work for you, not for the company.

❑ You do not have an ongoing, continuing relationship with the company.

❑ You set your own work hours.

❑ You can work less than full-time if you prefer.

❑ You do not have to work at the company's facilities.

❑ You are not required to follow a sequence of procedures established by the company.

❑ You do not have to submit progress reports on your work.

❑ You are paid by the job (number of massages), rather than by the hour, week, or month.

❑ You have to bear the cost of any travel or other expenses required to carry out the work.

❑ You use your own supplies and equipment; the company does not pay for them.

❑ You have invested in (paid for) any equipment or facilities you use.

❑ You assume a risk of loss if something goes wrong.

❑ You work for more than one company.

❑ You offer massages to the general public.

❑ The company cannot fire you; it can only decide whether to contract with you again in the future.

❑ If you fail to perform the services contracted for, the company could hold you legally liable.

The more boxes you checked, the more likely the IRS will agree that you are an independent contractor, meaning you are self-employed. If only a few of these statements apply to you, however, you may not meet the legal standard for being an independent contractor (even if you have signed a contract that says you are not an employee). Because the IRS considers you to be an employee, you should either change your work arrangements or have the organization(s) with which you have a contract withhold employment taxes.

For more information, go to Internal Revenue Service at www.irs.gov/tax. To request a ruling from the IRS whether an individual is an independent contractor or an employee, file IRS form SS-8, which can be downloaded from the IRS web site, or call 1-800-829-3676.

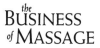

© 2002 American Massage Therapy Association, Evanston, IL. *The Business of Massage.* All Rights Reserved. 20026

On Your Own or with Other Owners?

If you have decided on self-employment, whether as an independent contractor who travels to a few clients, the co-owner of a large practice, or something in between, think about how to structure the ownership of your practice. This decision depends partly on whether you will work as the sole owner of your practice or will share ownership with others.

Sole Proprietors

Most self-employed massage therapists operate as independent contractors and own their businesses as sole proprietors. The IRS calls this arrangement a sole proprietorship. It is the simplest form of business organization. Basically, if you provide a service and someone pays you, you have a sole proprietorship.

If you work by yourself, providing massage in exchange for payment, and you are not an employee, you are an independent contractor and a sole proprietor. "Independent contractor" describes your relationship with the party who pays you. It means you have (formally or informally) contracted to provide particular services, rather than to become an employee. "Sole proprietor" describes ownership; it means you are the only owner of your business—and you do have a business, even if it consists only of you, some stationery, and a box of business cards.

The simplicity of forming and operating a business is the main reason so many massage therapists operate sole proprietorships. As a sole proprietor, you can practice under your own name or select a name for your practice. You can set up a practice in a home office (assuming local laws permit it) or in an office space that you rent alone, with a staff, or with other professionals. Or you can be an independent contractor who travels to other facilities where you have contracted to perform services.

A sole proprietorship has disadvantages, too. Working alone can feel isolating, and, compared to other forms of business, you may find it relatively difficult or expensive to borrow money, especially if you have not kept meticulous records. In a legal sense, a sole proprietorship is not separate from the individual owner. Therefore, a massage therapist who sets up an office but fails to pay all the related bills will be personally liable. That is, creditors can seek payment from the therapist's personal assets.

Similarly, if someone falls and breaks a hip in a therapist's office, and the therapist lacks general liability insurance to cover the person's injury-related expenses, the person could sue the therapist, and the therapist could be required to pay from personal assets.

If this level of liability concerns you, seek advice from a legal professional who can counsel you on protecting yourself legally in your particular situation. Also, cultivate relationships with experienced massage therapists, who can act as mentors. They may be able to allay many of your concerns.

General liability insurance is usually included with membership in a professional association.

Partnerships and Corporations

For therapists eager to build large practices, a sole proprietorship may be too limiting. These massage therapists instead share ownership with others by forming some type of partnership or corporation.

A partnership is an association of two or more people in which they agree to operate a business as co-owners. To start the business, they sign a partnership agreement, register the business's name with the proper state authorities, and obtain a business license if required by law. As with a sole proprietorship, the partners are personally liable for debts of the practice.

A corporation is a legal organization whose assets and liabilities are separate from those of its owners. Each state has laws spelling out the requirements for setting up a corporation. These requirements will include filling out papers called articles of incorporation, electing at least a minimum number of officers, and obtaining an Employer Identification Number from the IRS.

The federal government recognizes several types of partnerships and corporations. "Types of Businesses" (figure 1.9, page 35) shows the major types. If you are interested in forming any type of partnership or corporation, seek qualified legal and financial advice. Your advisers can help ensure that you satisfy all the legal requirements and structure the organization in a way that meets the objectives of all participants.

The success of any partnership or corporation will depend on the talent and commitment of all the owners. Remember, the time to evaluate your partners is before you sign the partnership agreement or articles of incorporation.

To assess whether a partnership relationship will benefit you, answer these questions about your prospective partner:
1. What talents and other resources will this person contribute to the practice?
2. What characteristics of this person will make him or her hard for me to get along with? Am I willing to work with the things I do not like?
3. Does the person really have access to the financial resources he or she has promised to contribute?
4. Will this person work the hours necessary to make the practice a success?
5. Does this person have a good track record of honoring promises and commitments?
6. Are this person's goals for the practice consistent with my own?
7. Does this person live up to my own standards professionally, ethically, and in terms of business sense?

Only when you are satisfied with your answers to all these questions should you form the partnership or corporation. It is much more difficult and costly to change your mind after you have entered into an agreement.

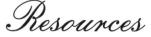

Information About Forming a Corporation or Partnership
- Ask your accountant or attorney.
- Go to the office of your state's secretary of state or corporate commission. (See the state government listings in your phone book or on their Web sites.)
- Small Business Administration: 1-800-8-ASK-SBA; www.sba.gov
- Sohnen-Moe Cherie, "Legal Structure," *Massage Therapy Journal,* Summer 1998.

Figure 1.9   Types of Businesses

Sole Proprietorship

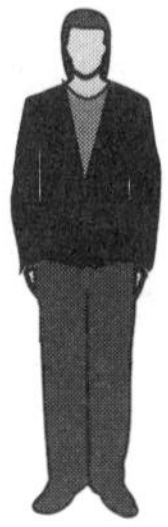

Sole Proprietorship:
- One person has ownership and liability

Partnership

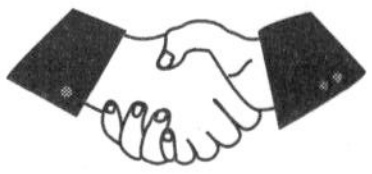

General Partnership:
- Partners share ownership and liability

Limited Partnership:

There are two types of partners in a Limited Partnership:
- General partners play an active role and have unlimited liability
- Limited partners invest in the partnership, do not play an active role, and have liability only up to the amount of their investment

Limited Liability Company (LLC):
- Permitted in most states: generally must have at least 2 owners
- Taxed as a partnership
- Owners' liability limited as in a corporation

Corporations

Articles of Incorporation

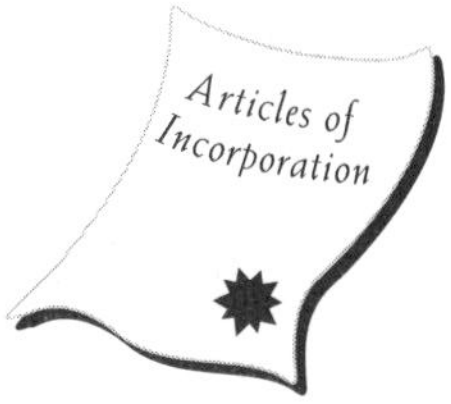

Corporation (sometimes called C Corporation):
- Separate entity from its owner, or stockholders, formed in accordance with state regulations
- Business pays income tax, and owners pay tax on any dividends

S Corporation (or Subchapter S Corporation):
- Corporation that meets IRS size and stock ownership requirements (if the corporation is small enough, a shareholder with at least 50% of the stock may request S corporation status)
- Pays taxes as a partnership
- Retains liability advantages of corporations

Professional Corporation:
- Separate entity from individual owners
- Taxed at higher rate than other corporations
- Limited liability for owners

Know Your Career Will Evolve

Most practitioners who have practiced massage therapy or bodywork for many years have seen their practices evolve from one type of business emphasis to another. This could happen for a variety of reasons:

- As a result of taking continuing education, they have discovered a specialty area that interests them, and would like to change the focus of their practice.

- Their clients have changed as the community around them has changed. Maybe new businesses have opened near their practice, and they now have the opportunity to develop an on-site seated-chair massage business. They might or might not want to carry the costs of keeping their private practice open if they are spending more of their time on-site at client locations.

- They have refined their skills as a massage therapist and have developed the stamina to handle a reasonable client load as an employee, and now they have the confidence to start their own private practice. Now that they are no longer as consumed with learning to refine their skills, they have the time to invest in learning the business aspects of operating their own practice.

- Their partner has been transferred to a new city, and in choosing to move there they no longer have an established client base. They decide to accept a position as a massage therapist employee.

- After many years as a practitioner, many of their clients have given them feedback that they would like to become massage therapists themselves, and the practitioner knows that their clients' choice is partly due to them being a role model. The practitioner decides that they would like to keep a few of their long-standing clients but also become an educator of massage therapists.

- They were a medical practitioner before they added massage therapy credentials to their repertoire, and now they would like to expand their contribution to include research, either as a participant or as a researcher.

- Their years of success as a practitioner and educator have motivated them to write articles for massage therapy publications and complementary and alternative medicine publications. They would also like to be a speaker at professional conferences and at training seminars.

All of these possibilities keep your future outlook on the profession of massage therapy and bodywork as exciting as your present one. No two individual career paths are the same.

Chapter Summary

As a new massage therapist, you are about to embark on a profession that offers a broad variety of career options. Many experienced practitioners recommend that you work as an employee for several years before opening your own business, although examples exist of individuals experienced in business and marketing who were successful in operating their own businesses as soon as they became licensed as massage therapists.

There are many ways you can choose how to start your career, such as taking self-assessment personality and interest inventories and working with a mentor. In deciding how to launch your career, consider carefully how your beliefs, attitudes, and values will affect your preferences.

If you decide to become self-employed, you will need to determine whether to structure your business as a sole proprietorship, a partnership, or a corporation. If you work at another business site, you will do so either as an employee of that business or as an independent contractor, which is a form of self-employment. It is important for tax purposes that you understand the distinction between being an employee and an independent contractor.

Significant trends that affect your career opportunities include growth in consumer acceptance and visibility of massage therapy, increasing interest in alternative health care, and increased research into the efficacy of massage. As more research in the areas of complementary and alternative health therapy is completed, consumers who rely on scientific measurement of health benefits will be more willing to try massage, and insurance companies might be more willing to include it as a covered benefit for their subscribers.

Career opportunities exist primarily in the fields of medical massage, spas, wellness programs, and in the fitness/sports area. Some practitioners also develop specialties in such areas as massage for pregnant women, infants, animals, or elderly persons.

No matter what you decide when you first complete your training as a massage therapist, you may be sure that your career will continue to grow and to change. The profession of massage therapy offers an abundance of career opportunities for experienced practitioners to expand their careers, just as it offers many opportunities to the beginning professional.

Review Questions

1. What are the pros and cons of starting your career as: a) self-employed; b) working first as an employee?

2. What tools can you use to help identify your needs, behaviors, beliefs and attitudes as they relate to your choice of career path?

3. How do your personal and cultural values, attitudes, and ethics influence your choice of career path?

4. What are significant trends that affect career opportunities in the profession of massage therapy and bodywork?

5. How does increased research of complementary and alternative therapies affect the profession of massage therapy?

6. What are primary areas of opportunity for working in the massage therapy profession?

7. What characteristics distinguish an independent contractor from an employee?

8. For what reasons would you choose to structure your business as a sole proprietorship vs. a corporation?

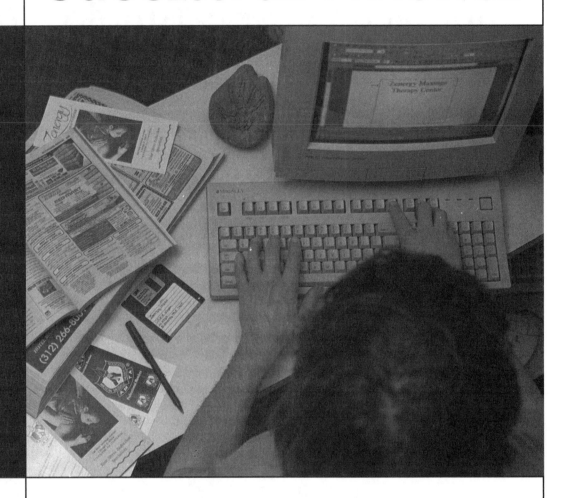

2

LAUNCHING *a* SUCCESSFUL PRACTICE

WHEN YOU GIVE YOUR FIRST MASSAGE FOR PAY, YOU BECOME A BUSINESSPERSON.

LAY THE GROUNDWORK THAT WILL CATAPULT YOU TO SUCCESS.

Chapter Objectives

1. Identify an appropriate sequence of steps for launching your massage career.

2. Create effective strategy and tools for job hunting.

3. Identify the components of a business plan.

4. Learn effective communications strategies to help you build a practice.

5. Identify common legal issues that you need to know when opening your practice.

In the previous chapter, you gained a broad perspective on the scope of business opportunities for massage therapists, and you examined how your individual attributes and interests will influence your choice of practice types. In this chapter you will learn about the specific steps required to bring to fruition the type of practice you want to have.

Employee *vs.* Self-Employed

What does it mean to have a practice? Whether you choose to provide massage as an employee, or as a self-employed massage therapist, you have a practice. Having a practice means that you create or choose an environment in which you practice your skills as a massage therapist in such a way that benefits your clients. How you do that, and with which clients, depends on the practice you choose.

This chapter helps you lay the foundation for building the type of practice you want. It presents a framework for creating a business plan, which can apply equally whether you're building your practice within the framework of being an employee or as a self-employed practitioner. It provides information about developing goals and objectives, also a skill that applies equally to being an employee or self-employed. The skills and requirements that are specific to being an employee, such as job-hunting and résumé writing, are presented separately from those required for being self-employed.

Your Practice as an Employee

As an employee, many elements of your practice are already established for you. The physical location already exists, and the client category—spa, sports/fitness, medical, wellness—will be determined by the type of business that employs you. Policies are already in existence.

Even within your employer's business, you will imprint your own identity on your individual practice. You will do this in your professional behavior toward the business that employs you and toward the clients you serve, as well as toward the new clients that you attract to the business. Your identity will come through in the way you greet people and in the way you follow up with them after the appointment, always working within the policies of your employer. Your identity will be further established by the ways in which you promote your employer's image.

As an employee, your interpersonal communication skills will be as important to you as your technical massage skills are. You will have the advantage of focusing on your skills as a massage therapist—your hand skills, your posture and biomechanic skills, your therapeutic relationship skills, and your stamina—while also learning your employer's business practices. As an employee, you will need to be flexible to accommodate your employer's business needs, which might include such things as receptionist duties or inventorying stock. But you will have the luxury of leaving many business details to your employer, such as employee payroll and building leases.

Your employer might or might not allow clients to specify an individual massage therapist for their sessions—but you want to conduct your practice within the employer's setting in such a way that clients would choose you if they could.

Your Practice as a Self-Employed Massage Therapist

If you become self-employed, many options are open to you. You may choose to establish an office in your home, you may become an independent contractor and provide massage in shared office space with another business, you may provide on-site massage at employee worksites, or you may go to your clients' homes to give massage. Or you may establish an independent practice, with leased space, and employ other massage therapists. You will have many decisions to make in choosing a location, planning the physical environment, and establishing policies. You will control the identity of your practice through such things as advertising, your business logo, your marketing plans, your physical place of business, and your policies regarding client service. Your attention to business details will be as important as your skills as a massage therapist are.

Professional Credentials

Whether you want someone to hire you, be your client, or lend you money, you want to be able to demonstrate that you are a professional. One way is with professional credentials. Credentials are accepted statements from a credible authority saying you are qualified to give massages. Credentials convey trustworthy information about the level of your competence. For clients, they also signal that you will provide reliable care.

Because there are important distinctions between one type of credential and another, the concept of credentials can be confusing. When you see a massage therapist's business card, you might see the person's name followed by a string of initials, such as LMT, AMTA, NCTMB. Here is a brief guide to help you understand the type of credentials you might want or need as a massage therapist.

Licensure
Municipalities and states have different licensing and/or regulatory requirements for massage therapists. Check with your local regulatory agency to find out the requirements that apply to you. (Licenses may also apply to your place of business, but these are not the same as professional licenses required for individuals.)

Certification
Certified means that you have met the requirements of an organization that tests applicants on a core body of knowledge in ethical and professional practices. For example, many states recognize the National Certification for Therapeutic Massage and Bodywork (NCTMB) credential. This credential is given when participants pass an exam administered by NCBTMB (National Certification Board for Therapeutic Massage and Bodywork), as well as meet standards for

Shared Wisdom
"Do the math: After adding up the amount per month you would be paying as a percentage to a clinic, you will see that it is possible to pay rent on your own office space. (For example, in a 60/40% split that is usual in a clinic type establishment, 40% on a $45 massage = $18 x 20 massages per week—considered full-time = $360 per week x 4 weeks in a month = $1,440 paid per month to the establishment out of *your* income.) In your own practice, you receive the entire $45, and the rent you would pay on office space would usually be much less than $1,440."

—*Laurie McCuistion, Licensed Massage Therapist, Magna, Utah*

ongoing education and recertification every four years. Some states have their own certification requirements. See the Continuing Education section in chapter 8 for more information about ongoing requirements to maintain certification.

School Certificates and Diplomas

Institutions and programs of massage therapy award certificates, or confer diplomas, to students upon successful completion of their curriculums. Most certificates and diplomas indicate the number of hours the student has completed in professional training.

Registered

Some states in the United States require that massage therapy practitioners be registered in order to legally use the term "massage therapist" on their business cards and in their business.

In Canada, registration is a credential that meets accepted standards in the health-related fields. It defines a body of knowledge common to all who are registered. Most provinces require a minimum 2,200 hours of training; British Columbia requires a minimum 3,000 hours. Some provinces use Canada's registration standards as their licensing examination, which in some cases opens the door for reciprocity between provinces. As of 2002, two provinces require registration status in order to practice massage therapy, and all provinces require registration status in order to secure insurance. Practitioners must renew registrations periodically as required by the governing agency.

Membership in a Professional Association

There are many professional associations that offer membership to eligible practitioners. The primary professional organizations at the national level are the American Massage Therapy Association (AMTA), a not-for-profit member-driven association, and the Associated Bodywork and Massage Professionals (ABMP) and International Massage Association (IMA), for-profit massage therapist/bodyworker organizations. When designating that you are a member of AMTA, you must include your category of membership, such as Professional Member of AMTA or Associate Member of AMTA. Professional associations also exist at local, state, and regional levels, and specific to many modalities. See Chapter 8 for a description of benefits you can derive from being a member of an organization with your professional peers.

Accreditation

Accreditation applies only to institutions, not to individuals. It means that the institution has met particular standards established by an accrediting organization. Accreditation must be renewed periodically to assure continued compliance with standards.

Using Abbreviations

Abbreviations such as LMT are great when you're communicating with your peers in the profession, but most clients will not be familiar with what they mean. If you are a licensed massage therapist, whenever possible spell out Licensed Massage Therapist on your business cards, letterhead, and other documents that clients see.

The National Certification Board for Therapeutic Massage and Bodywork specifies that individuals use the letters NCTMB following the name of the certified practitioner. The credential NCTMB stands for Nationally Certified Therapist of Massage and Bodywork. For clarity, when space allows, you might want to spell out "Nationally Certified in Therapeutic Massage and Bodywork."

Shared Wisdom
"Do one thing daily to further your career goal. Broken down this way, the tasks won't be overwhelming, yet you will be constantly and steadily moving toward your goal."

—*Pam Shelline, Sensory Development Institute, St. George, Utah*

Business Plans

Creating a business plan is your first step toward earning a living as a massage therapist. Putting your career goals and operational plans into writing is important whether you plan to be self-employed, or work as an employee for someone else. A business plan helps you define your goals and evaluate realistically whether or how those goals can be achieved. It helps you look at the immediate and near-term future as well as plan ahead for where you want to be in five years. If you plan to borrow money to fund your business's start-up, your lending institution will require a written business plan.

A written business plan will be important to you for two reasons: 1) you will need the documentation if you are going to request assistance from external sources, such as applying for a business loan, and 2) there is more financial investment and risk associated with starting your own business than in being an employee, so you want to be as thorough as possible in laying the groundwork before you open your doors.

The exercise of writing a business plan even if you do not plan to open a private practice immediately is still helpful because it makes you think about many aspects of your practice from the viewpoint of the owner. As an employee, your ability to wear the hat of the business owner will make you a real asset.

At the end of this chapter you will find the "Career and Practice Planning Worksheet" (figure 2.24, page 102), which provides the basis for a business plan. If you plan to borrow money, the lending institution you use might require its own business plan format. The resources box, "Sources of Information on Business Plans," lists several sources of business plan samples and guidelines.

You will refer to the "Career and Practice Planning Worksheet" throughout this textbook. Much of the information required to complete the worksheet is contained in this chapter. Other chapters provide more detailed information that will allow you to expand and refine your business plan, as you learn more.

Your first business plan step is to define your career goals and objectives.

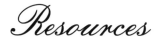

Sources of Information on Business Plans

- Abrams, Rhonda M. *The Successful Business Plan: Secrets and Strategies*. Grants Pass, OR: The Oasis Press, 1993.
- Canada BC Business Service Centre: www.sb.gov.bc.ca/smallbus/workshop/busplan.html
- Home BizNet, a Web site specializing in resources for home businesses: www.homebiznet.net
- Inc.com: www.inc.com/advice/writing_a_business_plan/
- NOLO Law for All: www.nolo.com/encyclopedia
- Service Corps of Retired Executives (SCORE), a free consulting service provided by the SBA: see the government listings in your phone book for the local office or visit www.score.org
- Small Business Administration (SBA), a federal agency that offers many publications and loan guarantee programs: 1-800-8-ASK-SBA or www.sba.gov
- SBA Business Plan Outline: www.sba.gov/starting/indexbusplans.html

Setting Goals and Objectives

Yogi Berra, a famous baseball player and coach who is equally famous for his comic wisdom, offered sage advice regarding the practice of setting goals and objectives when he said, "You've got to be very careful if you don't know where you're going, because you might not end up there." The beauty of setting goals and objectives is that they give you a roadmap that clearly marks the beginning, planned route, and final destination of your business journey. Setting goals helps you plan where you want to end up.

In determining what you want to achieve over the course of your career, you will create goals and objectives:

1. Goals are broad statements that express values or mission.
2. Objectives are more specific business-oriented statements in support of your goals. They are time-bound and measurable. That is, they are stated in terms of specifically what will happen, and when.

Goals can include both philosophical and practical statements. One way to develop goals is to answer questions such as the following:
- What kind of work do you want to do?
- Do you want to work alone or with others?
- What kind of business relationship do you want with others (as employer/employee or as partners)?
- What level of income do you want?
- For what do you want to be known?

Your goals might be stated in several different subject areas. Examples of different types of goals include:

Type of goal	Example
Short-term	Build up stamina to provide six massage sessions in one day
Long-term (five years)	Develop a specialty in infant massage
Financial	Pay back school loans
Personal	Flexibility to take up to six weeks off per year without pay
Client Profile	Wellness clients who are interested in learning how to optimize their health
Employer Profile	Medical massage practice with excellent reputation among oncology practitioners

To develop objectives, you would answer questions like the following, which should be relative to your goals:
- What steps do I need to take to achieve my goals?
- In what timeframe do I need or want to do certain things?
- How will I know if I have met my goals? This refers to putting measurements in place so you can keep track of how close you are to reaching your goals.

Objectives that would support the first goal shown above might be as follows:
Goal
Build up stamina to provide six massage sessions in one day.

Objectives
1. Within one month of graduation, get a job with a business that does a high volume of massage business.
2. Supplement my paid massages with two volunteer massages per week.

Finding a Job

Finding employment as a massage therapist could be as simple as answering an ad in the classified section of your local newspaper, interviewing for the position, and starting to work. But if you want a satisfying career, you'll want to devote careful thought about what your ideal job would be before you apply to any ads.

Often, the people who plan their job searches as an exercise in self-knowledge and self-marketing are those who land the best jobs. Before you create your résumé, know what your career goals are. You might already have a good idea of your goals. When it comes to money, for instance, there's probably a minimum amount that you must earn to cover your expenses. The more elusive goals, such as your long-term goals, might be harder to describe. These are the goals that will probably add the most satisfaction to your job hunt. If you make the mental and emotional commitment now to explore how you want your massage therapy training to make a difference to you and to others long-term, chances are you will be more selective in targeting a job.

Knowing your long-term goals allows you the flexibility to choose even those jobs that are not your ideal choices, because you can appreciate how certain aspects of the job are indeed helping you reach long-term goals. For instance, let's say your career dream is to open a private practice that employs four massage therapists and specializes in providing massage therapy to hospice patients and their families. But let's say the only job opportunity available right now is as a spa employee whose clients want primarily relaxation massage. As an employee of the spa, keeping your long-term goal in mind allows you to appreciate the spa because you are learning skills there that are transferable to your dream job in these ways:

1. You learn how to communicate with clients in a way that puts them at ease even if they are having a bad day.
2. You develop self-care skills within the context of performing a job that is sometimes stressful.
3. You observe from your employer the things you will do the same when you are an employer, and things you will do differently.
4. You welcome the opportunity to represent your employer as a provider of volunteer massage at events that benefit the type of organization you want to support.
5. You volunteer to speak to community groups about the benefits of massage, because you know that public speaking skills will benefit you now and in the future.
6. You invest your continuing education time and money in courses that help you reach your long-term goals.

Be choosy about selecting potential employers. You want your first work experience to be a positive one. It can be helpful to complete the "Potential Employer Profile" (figure 2.1, page 47) as you make your job-hunting decisions.

Figure 2.1

POTENTIAL EMPLOYER PROFILE WORKSHEET

Page 1 of 2

Number, in order of preference, the types of business you would most enjoy being associated with as a massage therapist (1 = first choice; 8 = last choice):

__ Fitness/Sports   __ Chiropractic office   __ Hospital

__ Massage therapy office   __ Physical therapy office   __ Other (describe)

__ Wellness center   __ Spa/Resort/Salon   _____

Identify two such businesses, based on your first and second choices above, within reasonable commute from your home:

(A) _____   (B) _____

Business A

Name of business: _____

Address: _____

Phone:_____   Owner/Manager:_____

Legal Form: ❑ Private   ❑ Franchise   ❑ Branch Office   ❑ Other

Years in business:_____   Years at present location:_____

Type(s) of massage offered: _____

Reputation in the community: _____

Target markets for this business:

   Age range: _____   Gender: _____

   Occupations: _____   Income: _____

   Educational level: _____   Openness to alternative therapies: yes/no

   Social/cultural environment: _____

1. How could this business benefit from incorporating your services? (For example, would you attract a younger clientele? Would you offer particular skills to athlete clients?) _____

2. What suggestions could you present to the owner of this business that would promote your presence in the business? _____
   _____

3. What do you anticipate your compensation would be from this business relationship?

   Salary range: _____

   Benefits (medical insurance, paid time off, etc.): _____
   _____

4. Other than income, what value would you seek from this working relationship? _____
   _____

the
BUSINESS
of MASSAGE

© 2002 American Massage Therapy Association, Evanston, IL. *The Business of Massage.* All Rights Reserved. #20026

Business B

Name of business: _____

Address: _____

Phone: _____ Owner/Manager: _____

Legal Form: ❑ Private ❑ Franchise ❑ Branch Office ❑ Other

Years in business: _____ Years at present location: _____

Type(s) of massage offered: _____

Reputation in the community: _____

Target markets for this business:

    Age range: _____ Gender: _____

    Occupations: _____ Income: _____

    Educational level: _____ Openness to alternative therapies: yes/no

    Social/cultural environment: _____

1. How could this business benefit from incorporating your services? (For example, would you attract a younger clientele? Would you offer particular skills to athlete clients?) _____
_____

2. What suggestions could you present to the owner of this business that would promote your presence in the business? _____

3. What do you anticipate your compensation would be from this business relationship?

    Salary range: _____

    Benefits (medical insurance, paid time off, etc.): _____
_____

4. Other than income, what value would you seek from this working relationship? _____
_____

Adapted from: Kiné-Concept Institute Business Success Workbook. Used by permission.

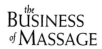

© 2002 American Massage Therapy Association, Evanston, IL. *The Business of Massage.* All Rights Reserved. #20026

Create Your Résumé

The purpose of your résumé is to let prospective employers know your qualifications for employment. In most cases, the employer will see your résumé before he or she has had the opportunity to meet you in person. Naturally, you want to make sure that your résumé and cover letter create a favorable impression.

The categories of information that are generally included on a résumé are:

Your name, address, telephone, and e-mail address

Summary of who you are and what you are seeking
This can be stated either as "Profile" information, which summarizes your strengths and skills, or as an "Objective," which states the type of position you are seeking.

Qualifications
List your credentials and describe the modalities you are qualified to practice. Graduates of 500-hour programs are usually qualified to practice Swedish techniques. Most other modalities require additional training and additional certificates of completion. For information on credentials, see the section "Professional Credentials" earlier in this chapter.

Education
List schools you have attended (high school and beyond) and any workshops or seminars that are relevant to the type of position you are seeking.

Employment history
Name and location of employer, dates of employment, short description of job, and anything about your experience there that applies to the type of position you are seeking.

Awards and affiliations
List your membership in a professional association and any awards or professional-related affiliations that a prospective employer might be interested in. For instance, as a student, did you ever give a presentation about the benefits of massage to fitness club members at the YMCA? While you are a student is a good time to do things that will help you on your résumé.

Many job ads specify "previous experience required." But what if you are just graduating from massage therapy training, and you don't have previous massage therapy job experience? Learn how to translate previous job experiences or volunteer experiences into skills that will help you in your job search. Even if you've never before held a job as a massage therapist, consider how the following experiences would sound to a potential employer:

- As a student intern, I provided more than 175 massages to clients through supervised student clinic. I developed a 20% rate of return clients, which was higher than the class average.
- My previous job as veterinary technician taught me the importance of customer service skills and putting people at ease who are under stress.

Select your examples carefully, so you can limit your résumé to one page (or two, if you have extensive experience that is applicable). See "Sample Résumé" (figure 2.2, page 50) as an example.

Figure 2.2

JAN A. SANGER
1234 Any Street
Anywhere, USA
(555) 555-5555
jsanger@email.com

OBJECTIVE

To develop a professional, ethical, client-oriented and therapeutic massage career.

QUALIFICATIONS

Education from COMTA accredited massage therapy school
- Effective and ethical delivery of massage therapy
- Proficiency in S.O.A.P charting and documentation
- Knowledge of massage indications and contraindications
- Understanding of physiological developmental stages
- Current Red Cross certification in CPR & First Aid Safety

AMTA Professional Member

EXPERIENCE

SCHOOL OF NATURAL THERAPEUTICS, Anywhere, WI
Student – 9/00 to 6/01
- 650 hours classroom/coursework
- 150 hours of clinical practice in student clinic

MUTUAL INSURANCE COMPANY, Anywhere, WI
Commercial Policy Processing Technician – 3/95 to 9/00
- Reviewed and prepared commercial policies and set up yearly renewal files
- Coordinated underwriting information and processed new business applications

LIFE INSURANCE COMPANY OF AMERICA, Anywhere, ME
Sales Support Representative – 12/92 to 3/95
- Prepared underwriting data (financial and medical)
- Ordered medical exams, blood tests, and physician statements
- Supported brokers with product information, customer feedback, and new business leads

Selected for special assignments:
- Designed office personnel grid for use in field offices
- Awarded 1995 "Rep of the Year Award" based on increased territory sales

Customer Service Billing Representative – 9/87 to 12/92
- Maintained ongoing accounts and premium payments
- Processed reconciliation of client accounts and responded to client requests
- Served as backup supervisor within work region
- As accounting point person, advised coworkers on proper accounting methods

Selected for special assignments:
- Managed several field offices; encouraged teamwork to ensure that all deadlines were met
- Designed biweekly schedule for flex-time employees

EDUCATION

School of Natural Therapeutics
Anywhere, Wisconsin
800 hour Massage Therapy Program – 2001

Maine College
Anywhere, Maine
B.S., Business Administration/Marketing – 1987

REFERENCES

Available upon request

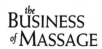
the
BUSINESS
of MASSAGE

© 2002 American Massage Therapy Association, Evanston, IL. *The Business of Massage.* All Rights Reserved. #20026

Create Cover Letters

Letters are one of the most important tools you can use in your job search. You will direct letters to advertised job ads as well as to contacts that you hope have jobs or suggestions you might be interested in. Your cover letter reflects your personality and allows you to pique the prospective employer's interest to learn more about you. Your cover letter will be tailored to fit each opportunity.

A cover letter should not take the place of personal contact. After sending a letter, follow up with a phone call to say you'd like to visit the place of business and to stop by to meet the prospective employer in person.

- Every cover letter will include an introduction, a body, and a close. The introduction is where you introduce yourself and catch the reader's interest. This is where you would mention the person who referred you, if appropriate.

- The body of the letter describes how you are suited for the job. Motivate the reader to want to meet you by describing how your skills can help the prospective employer's organization.

- The close is your final paragraph. Tell the prospective employer that you will call next week to request an appointment for an interview. Express your appreciation for his or her time and interest.

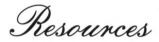

Sources of Job Leads
- other massage therapists
- mentors and friends
- schools with massage training programs
- Search the Web for "jobs" + "massage therapy." Depending on your targeted clientele, you might search on "jobs" + "health care" or "wellness" or "spas" or "fitness club"
- AMTA Job Network (available to members at www.amtamassage.org)
- professional publications such as *Massage Therapy Journal* and *Massage Magazine*
- newsletters from professional organizations and their regional chapters
- classified ads in local newspapers

Communication Strategies for Interviewing

When you interview for a job, be prepared to present your qualifications and to answer questions about your career goals. Practice your responses with a friend or your mentor. Review your résumé, and anticipate questions your potential employer might ask. Think through how your previous job experience, if not as a massage therapist, gave you skills that are transferable to a massage therapy job.

Practicing your responses with a friend might seem awkward, but it is well worth the time. Even if you are confident of your qualifications, speaking about them out loud isn't always as easy as it seemed in your head. And if you are not sure how you would answer questions where you don't feel confident —a lack of experience, previous long or numerous periods as unemployed, responding to a question you know a potential employer is not allowed by law to ask—it will help you tremendously to practice before you are in the actual interview.

For instance:

Situation	Possible response
Lack of experience	"Even though this will be my first paid employment as a massage therapist, our student internships were very comprehensive in giving me actual experience with clients and with business practices such as scheduling appointments and collecting payments." —or—"My previous employment as [...] gave me good experience in providing customer satisfaction, plus I learned good work habits that make me even more valuable as a massage therapist—things like punctuality, reliability and knowing how to work efficiently in an office environment."
Periods of unemployment	Be open about the reason for unemployment and explain that the condition for previous unemployment has now changed. "Now that my education, skills, and schedule put me in a good position to work full-time as a massage therapist, I'm eager to participate in a practice where I can benefit people."
If asked an inappropriate or illegal question	Be direct and firm, but not antagonistic, in rephrasing the interviewer's question to you in appropriate terms, such as: "I believe that, in asking that question, you are trying to understand whether I can be relied upon to work the hours required. You will find that I am very reliable because I place a high priority on getting repeat business, and I want clients to know they can depend on me to keep my appointments." If the interviewer persists in asking inappropriate questions, you should feel free to say, "Maybe you are not aware that the question you are asking me is not allowed by law. If I can answer other questions that pertain to the job you advertised, I would be happy to do so."

Be ready to ask the prospective employer questions to determine whether the job for which you are interviewing will help you achieve your career goals, such as:

- What kinds of clients do you have?
- What responsibilities does the job include? (Request a job description, if the organization has prepared one.)
- What are your policies for scheduling and tips?
- How many of the clients are insurance clients? (You may want this information because insurance companies may dictate the kind of massage therapy you provide. Are you willing to work within these limitations?)
- How does massage therapy fit into your organization's mission?
- What expectations would the business have of me? (Would you be expected to bring your own massage table to the workplace; provide your own oils/lotions or music; perform office duties?)

It is not unusual for a prospective employer to request a massage from the practitioner/job candidate. When you go to the interview, dress appropriately to allow for the potential of giving a massage. If appropriate, you may even volunteer to demonstrate your skills by offering a complimentary massage. Customize the massage to the type of job for which you're applying, such as whether it's sports/fitness or relaxation. Inquire about the interviewers' preferences in massage, as you would with a real client. See the boxed information, "Criteria for Interview Demo Massage," as a guide to criteria a prospective employer might use in evaluating the effectiveness of your massage.

Eventually, but perhaps not in the first interview, if you think the organization might be a good fit, you will want to know whether the job meets your earnings objectives. Therefore, you need to have in mind how much money you need to earn. Among AMTA members reporting full-time massage income in 2000, about a third earned between $30,000 and $50,000, and nearly a fifth earned over $50,000. You will want to make informal inquiries among friends and associates to find out what customary fees are, as well as what percentage of fees employers customarily take, in your locale. When you think about income, be realistic about understanding how much money will be taken out for taxes, and what your expenses will be (such as commuting or any supplies you might have to provide yourself).

Criteria for Interview Demo Massage

1. Pressure too light or too heavy
2. Temperature too cold or too warm
3. Comfort of headrest and bolster placements
4. Draping insufficient or awkward
5. Practitioner talked too much
6. Practitioner wasn't responsive to questions
7. Smooth transition between strokes

Consider whether you want to be paid a flat rate or a percentage of what the business charges for each massage session, if this is negotiable. Also ask about benefits such as health insurance, paid vacation time, and reimbursement of continuing education expenses. Review your potential employer's benefits package to see what kinds of insurance are included and whether you will be responsible for a portion of the premiums.

Always send a thank you letter to the person who interviewed you within 24 hours after the interview.

Job hunting can be educational because you can learn about the different settings that employ massage therapists and about the different modalities that tend to be used in various settings. Even if you do not think a particular interview will turn into a job offer, you can ask for a chance to meet with a person you think will have insights to share about a massage therapy career.

Once you have accepted a position, you might want to consider sending a note to individuals who gave you advice while you were job hunting, and always to those who gave you referrals. Even if a person's referral did not lead to your new job, you will want to express your appreciation for the help, and to inform the person of the job you selected. Maybe even enclose a few business cards if the person could be a source for referring clients to you at your new practice.

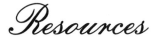

Advice on Job Hunting and Résumé Preparation
- Talk to practicing massage therapists to find out what they like and don't like about their practices. Find out what other jobs they have had as massage therapists, and what they did and didn't like about other jobs.
- Find a mentor who is willing to help you build your professional skills. Participate in professional associations and organizations, and take advantage of opportunities to build relationships where you can learn from someone who has more experience than you do.
- Read books and articles about job hunting.
- Ashley, Martin and Deborah Fay. *Massage: A Career at Your Fingertips* student workbook. Carmel, NY: Enterprise Publishing, 1999.
- Bolles, Richard N. *The 1999 What Color is Your Parachute? A Practical Manual for Job-Hunters and Career-Changers.* Berkeley: Ten Speed Press, 1999.
- Sohnen-Moe, Cherie. *Business Mastery, Third Edition.* Phoenix: Sohnen-Moe Associates, Inc., 1997.
- Helpful Web sites:
  AMTA Job Network: www.amtamassage.org/jobnet/home.htm
  www.jobweb.com
  www.questcareer.com
  www.free-résumé-tips.com

Starting Your Business

To establish your own business is a tremendous undertaking. Many experienced practitioners recommend that you work as an employee before you consider becoming self-employed. The advantages of this approach were discussed in chapter 1.

If or when you decide you want to establish your own business, you will want to prepare a formal business plan, as discussed at the beginning of this chapter. You may use the "Career and Practice Planning Worksheet" at the end of this chapter, or one of the many business-building toolkits available from the Small Business Administration or other resources listed on page 44. The worksheet follows the basic format of a business plan, so if you need to borrow money to set up a practice, you can also use it as the basis for preparing a loan application.

Background—Market Need

In the next part of your business planning, you will address the environment in which you plan to work, defining the needs that exist and how you hope to meet the needs you have identified. A key to success in establishing the level of market need, also known as demand, in your area is striking a healthy balance between your enthusiasm about the growth of massage therapy, and fear of too few clients. You want to be realistic—neither too optimistic nor pessimistic—about how many clients you can attract to your business. Reasons for enthusiasm include the increasing acceptance of alternative health therapies, increased third party insurance reimbursement for massage services (see "Client Insurance" section in chapter 3), and more research to prove the efficacy of massage (see "Research" section in chapter 8). For positive indicators about the growth of massage therapy, see "Consumer Survey Facts" (chapter 1, figure 1.2, page 12).

In addition, you will describe your qualifications, and the qualifications of others working with you, to meet those needs. As you start planning for your practice, this section will help you describe to others why they should choose you as a provider of massage. How do you differ from other practitioners in your area? What will attract clients to your business?

Estimating Supply and Demand

At the local level, your success as a massage therapist requires that your services meet a need in the market or community where you practice. Whether they will or not depends on the demand for massage and how well that demand is met already by other massage therapists. If the existing demand is less than the supply, consider how you can educate people about the benefits of massage and thus increase the demand for it, such as volunteering at community outreach events. See chapter 7 for strategies and tips on increasing demand and visibility.

By getting to know the local market in your community and surrounding areas, you identify the potential for your practice. This is a three-step process:

1. *Estimate current supply:* Estimate the number of practitioners already offering massage and whether they practice full-time or part-time. This tells you how much supply already exists in your community.
2. *Estimate total demand:* Estimate the demand for massage in your market— that is, the number of clients (massage consumers) in your area times the number of massage sessions you estimate they will get per year.
3. *Calculate unmet demand:* Subtract the current supply from the total demand. The remainder is the unmet demand. If the unmet demand is large enough to support your career goals, there is a good opportunity for you in the community you have chosen.

See "Consumer Survey Facts" (chapter 1, figure 1.2, page 12) for data about consumer growth trends in getting massages, or view the latest survey results at the American Massage Therapy Association Web site: www.amtamassage.org, and click on Massage Information Center. This site contains the latest consumer survey information as well as recent statistics regarding the demand for massage.

Estimating Supply

Look at the number of massage therapists currently serving your market's need for massage. Other massage therapists can help you build awareness of massage's benefits, but, of course, clients of theirs might not be clients of yours. You should be aware of other sources of massage in your community. Related professions might be considered secondary competition, such as chiropractors, physical therapists, or estheticians. In some cases you might collaborate with them to expand your mutual client bases, and in other cases their clients would not see a massage therapist in addition to seeing them.

"Estimating Supply" (figure 2.3, page 57) shows a process for doing this. It makes a few assumptions:
- Half of the massage therapists work full-time, giving an average of 24 hours of massage sessions per week. (More than 17 hours of actual massage sessions a week is considered full-time.)
- The other half give an average of 10 hours of massage sessions per week.
- All the massage therapists work 50 weeks per year.
- Clients receive eight massage sessions per year (the national average).

If you can estimate in which ways your community is different from the national average, you can adjust the numbers accordingly.

Figure 2.3 Estimating Supply

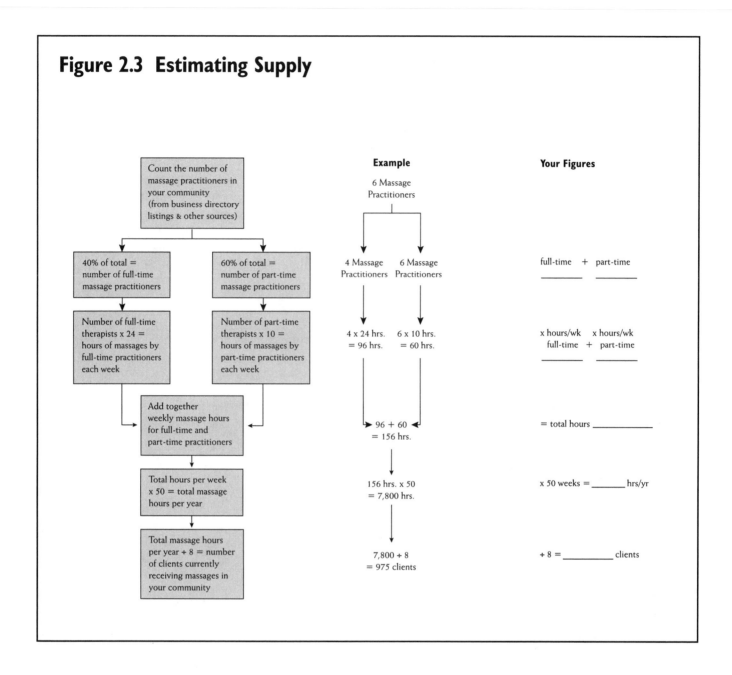

Estimating Demand in Your Area

If you know general or national patterns, you can begin to investigate the demand in your area, and how well that demand is being met already. For help in identifying national patterns, see "Consumer Survey Facts" (chapter 1, figure 1.2, page 12). The 17 percent of "adult Americans" cited in the study who received massage in the past year were adults living in private households. To estimate the number of people in that category where you live, you might ask your local library, city hall, chamber of commerce or business development to help you.

Do you expect local demand to be typical of the national average? If so, about 17 percent of the local adult population who live in private households would be potential clients of all the massage therapists in the area over a one-year period. A leading study reported that Americans who get massages average 8.4 visits a year [Eisenberg, et al. "Trends in Alternative Medicine Use in the United States, 1990-1997." *Journal of the American Medical Association* 280(18): 1569-1575, Nov. 11, 1998].

Using survey information and knowing national patterns can be helpful when you are trying to make estimates. Keep in mind that this is not an exact science, and there is no one formula that is going to give you the "right" answer. In addition to making a quantitative estimate, you will want to factor in anecdotal information, such as: How many people do you know personally who might be clients? How open are your community's residents to alternative health methods? Do you intend to open your business in an area that has a massage therapy school? (The assumption here would be that the supply of trained massage therapists could be higher than average in a town with a massage training school, versus in a town that does not have such a school.)

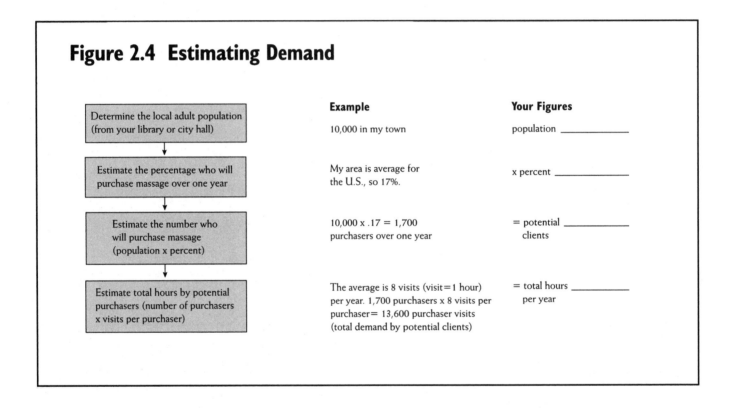

Figure 2.4 Estimating Demand

	Example	Your Figures
Determine the local adult population (from your library or city hall)	10,000 in my town	population _____
Estimate the percentage who will purchase massage over one year	My area is average for the U.S., so 17%.	x percent _____
Estimate the number who will purchase massage (population x percent)	10,000 x .17 = 1,700 purchasers over one year	= potential _____ clients
Estimate total hours by potential purchasers (number of purchasers x visits per purchaser)	The average is 8 visits (visit=1 hour) per year. 1,700 purchasers x 8 visits per purchaser= 13,600 purchaser visits (total demand by potential clients)	= total hours _____ per year

Unmet Demand

The potential for your practice is high if you estimate that the total demand for massage therapy is much greater than the number of clients already being served by practicing massage therapists. There should be enough unserved clients to keep you busy for the number of hours you want to spend giving massages. Here is how to determine the potential for your market:

1. *Supply:* Show your community's supply of total massage hours now provided by massage practitioners.
2. *Minus Demand:* Subtract the demand for massage hours from the number of supply hours.
3. *Unmet Demand in Hours:* The difference gives you the number of unmet demand hours.
4. *Unmet Demand in Number of Clients:* Divide unmet demand hours by eight (if you think the number of clients visits per year in your community is the same as the national average) to get the number of potential clients in your community.

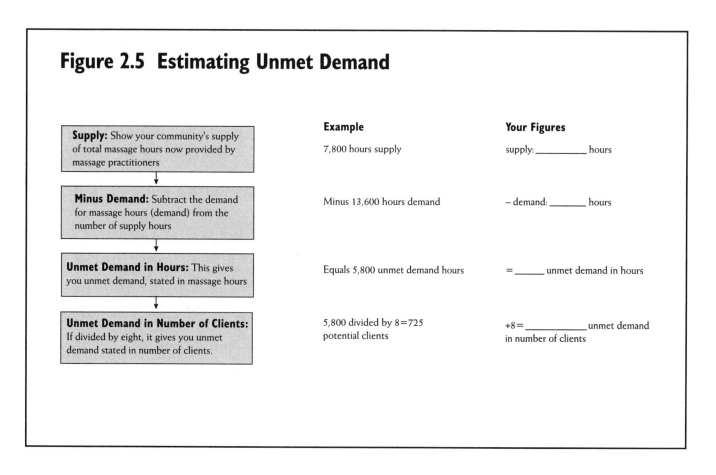

Figure 2.5 Estimating Unmet Demand

	Example	**Your Figures**
Supply: Show your community's supply of total massage hours now provided by massage practitioners	7,800 hours supply	supply: _____ hours
Minus Demand: Subtract the demand for massage hours (demand) from the number of supply hours	Minus 13,600 hours demand	– demand: _____ hours
Unmet Demand in Hours: This gives you unmet demand, stated in massage hours	Equals 5,800 unmet demand hours	= _____ unmet demand in hours
Unmet Demand in Number of Clients: If divided by eight, it gives you unmet demand stated in number of clients.	5,800 divided by 8 = 725 potential clients	÷ 8 = _____ unmet demand in number of clients

Your Potential

The next step is determining how many of those potential clients you want to attract to your business. This is estimating your individual supply of hours, as shown in "Estimating Your Potential" (figure 2.6, below). To do this, you would calculate how many massage hours you want to provide each week. Keep in mind that your work hours will be longer than your massage hours because of the time it takes to perform all the non-massage duties required to operate your business.

1. Hours you want to work each week
2. Times weeks you want to work each year
3. Divided by eight visits per client per year
4. Equals number of clients you need
5. Your Potential—Compare your supply to the unmet demand. If your supply is less than or equal to the unmet demand, your potential is promising. If your supply exceeds the unmet demand, you will have to expand the area you serve, choose a less-served area, or develop marketing and education strategies to increase the demand in your area. See chapter 7 for marketing strategies that can help you develop a plan.

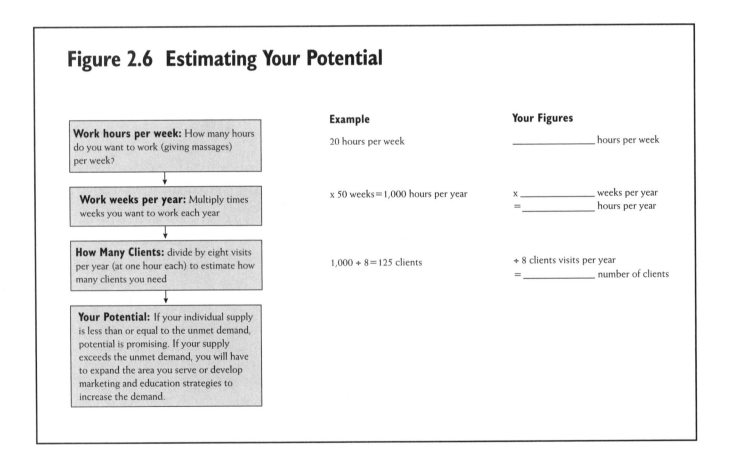

Figure 2.6 Estimating Your Potential

Work hours per week: How many hours do you want to work (giving massages) per week?

Work weeks per year: Multiply times weeks you want to work each year

How Many Clients: divide by eight visits per year (at one hour each) to estimate how many clients you need

Your Potential: If your individual supply is less than or equal to the unmet demand, potential is promising. If your supply exceeds the unmet demand, you will have to expand the area you serve or develop marketing and education strategies to increase the demand.

Example

20 hours per week

x 50 weeks = 1,000 hours per year

1,000 ÷ 8 = 125 clients

Your Figures

_____ hours per week

x _____ weeks per year
= _____ hours per year

÷ 8 clients visits per year
= _____ number of clients

If you live in an area where you feel confident that you will have as many clients to support your business as you need, or that you will be able to increase the number of clients through your marketing efforts, you are ready to develop the rest of your plan. The following section includes a brief overview of the areas you need to decide about marketing your business. For more detailed information about marketing, see chapter 7.

Marketing Objectives

In completing your "Career and Practice Planning Worksheet" (figure 2.24, page 102), you will describe your potential clients, your services and products, your pricing, and your communications plans. Answering the questions on the worksheet in each of these subject areas will help you develop specific marketing objectives. Objectives describe what you want to accomplish.

To write an objective, think about your goals and how you will measure what you want to achieve. Write a first draft. Then modify it so that it meets the criteria just listed. This is not as easy as it sounds, but careful planning will help you communicate your expectations to yourself and to others. They should be specific, time-bound and achievable. For example:

Good Example of Objective
Have a minimum of 15 active clients over age sixty-five within first 18 months of operation.

Not a Good Example of Objective
Get a more focused client base.

Build up to ten percent of clients who received third-party reimbursement by end of year.

Have clients who receive third-party reimbursement.

Growth rate of 25 percent the second year and 10 percent in third and fourth years.

Aggressive growth in second year and more moderate after that.

Marketing Strategy

The marketing strategy for your business describes how you will attract to your business the type of clients you intend to serve. Decision areas include what types of modalities your business will offer, the image you want to project, and whether and what types of products you will sell. After you determine your overall marketing strategy, you will have set the stage for deciding what marketing tactics you will use in carrying out your strategy—such as direct mail, volunteering at events, advertising, and other promotional techniques. See chapter 7 for more information about developing successful marketing strategies.

Clients

Almost anyone can benefit from therapeutic massage, but to plan to market your services to everybody is not practical. The next section of the worksheet asks you to target the categories of people you want to serve. Ask yourself whom you can approach to be a client, as well as who can refer clients to you. Figure 2.7 (page 62) identifies categories of potential clients, and chapter 7 provides details on identifying and marketing to these potential client categories.

You will need to find out whether you have targeted enough potential client categories to keep your practice busy.

Shared Wisdom

"Number One Rule: Don't quit your day job too soon! Once you have met your break-even point three months in a row, it is fairly safe to quit the day job and put all your energy into growing your business to full-time. Building a solid clientele requires time, because word-of-mouth is still the best marketing. Don't put yourself in the position of not being able to pay rent or buy groceries because you quit your day job before you had enough clients to support you."

—Peggy Smith, BMSI Institute, Overland Park, Kansas

Figure 2.7   Possible Client Categories for Massage Therapy

Adults seeking stress relief and relaxation

Adults seeking massage as preventive medicine or to enhance wellness

Healthcare patients

    Acute or chronic illnesses

    Recovery from illness or injury

    Pre- or postoperative care

    Hospice care (mostly volunteer)

    Recovery from trauma or abuse

Elderly adults (geriatric massage) (much is volunteer)

Pregnant Women

Infants

Children

Dancers and other performers (much is volunteer)

Athletes (sports massage)
    Sports teams
    Schools (mostly volunteer)
    Athletic centers and health clubs

Corporate and government organizations
    Chair massage for employees on-site
    Massages in corporate health facilities

Animals (horses, dogs, zoo residents, pets)

Your Services and Products

Next, define the range of services you want to offer. Some massage therapists like to focus on a particular modality of massage they enjoy performing. Others see massage as part of a wider range of related services they want to offer clients. (If so, they may have to meet additional qualifications to provide those services.) Yet others seek professional growth and enjoyment from teaching, research, and public education. If you want to do several of these, you will need to plan carefully the number of hours you will spend on giving massage sessions and other income-related activities, allowing enough time for your other professional activities.

Some practitioners also sell merchandise. According to 1998 research by AMTA, the products most frequently sold are oils, body lotions, aromatherapy products, and vitamins. Others sell CDs, books, jewelry, magnetic products, and T-shirts. If you want to do this, first consider how well the products fit within the scope of your practice. Do they support your image as a professional?

Before deciding to sell products, consider the drawbacks as well as the potential for profit. Liability issues might arise if a client is allergic to a particular oil or lotion, or if a client misuses a movement aid. Individuals can order products so inexpensively off the Internet that many product vendors are finding it difficult to make a profit unless they can order in bulk. If you buy a small quantity and keep your prices low, your profit disappears. Some practitioners feel that selling products detracts from their main focus, providing massage.

In some states, licensure for massage therapists prohibits the sale of products. Find out whether your state imposes such restrictions. If product sales are permitted and the products you want to offer are a good fit, plan for the expense of ordering the products, keeping them in stock, and maintaining adequate records of inventory and sales, including the collection of any sales tax.

Pricing

Whatever array of services and products you offer, you will need to make pricing decisions. Nationally, AMTA has found that the charge for a one-hour massage by a full-time massage therapist ranges from $45 to $75 (up to 30 percent more for an out-call, when you go to a client's home). See "Average Fees Charged by Massage Therapists Nationwide" (chapter 1, figure 1.5, page 14) for information on average fees for massages of various durations.

Keep in mind that what you charge per hour for massage times the number of hours you work is the total gross income from your practice, before all taxes and expenses. For example, if you charge $50 per hour, with 20 hours of actual massage sessions per week, your gross practice income (before expenses) for 50 weeks would be $50,000.

In setting your fees, consider your costs, as well as prices for comparable products and services from other sources. In general, conform to local pricing custom. If you charge more, clients may conclude you are too expensive. If you charge less, they may not value your services as highly. By charging less than the going rate, you will also soften the local market and thus make it more difficult long-term for you and your peers to charge fees that cover your expenses. Either way, you must then communicate why your services are a value or are worth more than similar services.

There are no official professional or ethical guidelines to follow that specify a stance on discounting. Many experienced massage therapists express strong opinions, pro and con, about the practice of discounting their services. Those in favor of it view it as a good promotional technique. They offer discounts to attract clients who see massage as a luxury they cannot afford but who might become regular clients if they actually experience the benefits of one. They offer volume discounts as a way of expressing gratitude to clients who get regular massages from them.

The other view of discounts is that massage therapy is a health benefit, and professionals do not offer their services at a discounted rate. Some massage therapists feel that the practice of discounting diminishes the professionalism of massage therapy. Offering a free massage to a client who has referred other clients to you, however, might be viewed as a thank-you or as a payment in lieu of advertising expenses.

Another aspect of discounting concerns whether you are willing to discount your fees in order to be included in insurance companies' or HMO's list of approved providers. The pros and cons of participating in these programs are extensive, and there is no clear "best practice" among massage therapists regarding participation. More information regarding becoming an approved healthcare provider for purposes of insurance reimbursement is discussed in chapter 3, in the section "Client Insurance," on page 149.

Communications

Image
Your practice's image is based on many factors: the name of your business; your business card and stationery; the size and style of signage; the section of the city you're in; the answering-machine message callers hear when you're not available to answer the phone (or is it a live answer?); the building your business is in; the furnishings in your reception area and in your practice rooms; your advertising.

As you choose every aspect of your business, keep your target client in mind. Ask yourself questions that apply to your particular business plan, such as:
Would this convey trust and credibility?
Would this help clients anticipate a soothing, relaxing environment?
Would this help me build a referral network with the medical community?

Naming Your Practice
Your massage therapy practice needs a name. You can use your own name or a name that describes your business in another way. Remember that this name will identify your services to the public. You will use it on your business cards, stationery, and checks; on any signs or brochures you have printed; when you answer the phone; and when you encourage people to refer potential clients to you.

Often, a massage therapist setting up independent contractor relationships with clients simply uses his or her own name as the name of the practice. For example, if Pat Fitzpatrick is Nationally Certified in Therapeutic Massage and Bodywork and is a Professional Member of AMTA, she can operate under the name Pat Fitzpatrick, NCTMB, Professional Member AMTA. That name would appear on her business cards and brochures, and on news releases she sends out describing workshops she will give. "Pros and Cons of Choosing Business Names" (figure 2.8, below), summarizes some pros and cons of using your own name for your practice.

You might also consider the advantages to choosing a name for your business that's at the beginning of the alphabet so your business appears at or near the top of business directory listings.

Figure 2.8:   Pros and Cons in Choosing Business Names

USING YOUR OWN NAME

Pros	*Cons*
simplicity	may not convey enough information about
personal assurance of putting your	your practice
reputation on the line	may not be suitable if you decide to expand practice

USING A FICTITIOUS OR ASSUMED NAME

Pros	*Cons*
protects name from misuse by others	creating name that is understandable and
conveys idea that practice is bigger than	unique may be a challenge
one practitioner	registering name may be more work than
can choose name that's easy to remember	using your own and it has a cost
or pronounce than your own name	may have to pay annual license fee
can use name that conveys benefits of	
having a massage	

Trade Names

If you form a partnership or corporation, you and your co-owners will have to agree on a name for the practice. Some sole practitioners also prefer to choose a trade name, which may be called a fictitious or assumed name. As noted in "Pros and Cons in Choosing Business Names" (figure 2.8, above), a made-up name may be more memorable or easier to pronounce than your own name. You may want to convey an image of the practice as more than just an individual giving massages. That image might be helpful, for example, when negotiating a lease for office space, because a landlord might be more impressed with what seems to be a bigger organization.

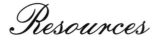

How to Avoid Trademark Conflicts When Registering a Web Domain Name

The Internet Corporation for Assigned Names and Numbers (ICANN) is a non-profit organization that provides domain name management. A domain name is the familiar name you see in Web site URLs that typically end in .com, .net, or .org. To learn about domain name administration, go to ICANN at www.icann.org.

To register a domain name, go to InterNIC at www.internic.net.

See chapter 7, "Electronic Presence" section, page 239, for more information about establishing Web sites.

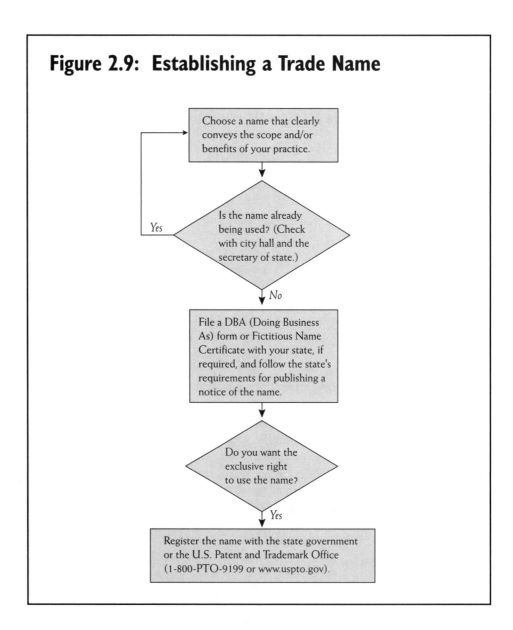

Figure 2.9: Establishing a Trade Name

The flowchart for "Establishing a Trade Name" (figure 2.9, page 66) provides basic directions for establishing a trade name, including the important step of researching to be sure no one already is using the name. A good place to start is with the U.S. Patent and Trademark Office Web site (www.uspto.gov), where, at no cost, you can search a database of trademarks. In Canada, each province has its own registration authority. You can search a database of trademarks through the Canadian Intellectual Property Office at www.strategis.ic.gc.ca.

Trade Names and Trademarks

The terms trade name and trademark have specific legal meanings. Your trade name is the name of your business (other than your own name). Your trademark, if you have one, would be some combination of a logo and words that separately or together identify your business. For example, you might select the trade name "Healing Hands," then design a logo of two hands surrounded by the practice's name. The image of the hands and the name would be your trademark.

Logos and Trademarks

When you have decided on a name, think about how you will communicate that name. Remember, every time people read the name on your stationery, business cards, signs, forms, or other printed materials, they will be reminded of you and your services. To send a consistent message about your business, your services, and your professionalism, you will want a well-designed logo. It could include the name of your business (which might be your own name) and could also incorporate a picture or other design elements.

If you are artistically inclined—especially if you know how to select type fonts and choose ink colors—you might want to design your own logo. However, keep in mind that an ability to draw is no substitute for experience in graphic design. The money you spend for the expertise of a graphic designer will be a good investment if the outcome is a well-designed logo that reinforces a professional, caring image. See guidelines discussed in this chapter for finding professional help.

Operations: Where and How You Will Practice

Where do you plan to work and what will you need in order to set it up? This section identifies the main categories of cost and policy considerations. More detailed information about the qualitative aspects of these categories is contained in chapters 4 and 5.

Selecting a Location

Like purchasing insurance, selecting a location is an essential part of getting started for every massage therapist. Location decisions fall into two basic categories:
- You must decide whether to set up a home office or a separate location.
- If you have decided to use a location other than your home, you need to select a space that is appropriate for your business.

"Practice Time Spent at Different Locations" (figure 2.10, page 68) summarizes where AMTA members, on average, spend most of their work time.

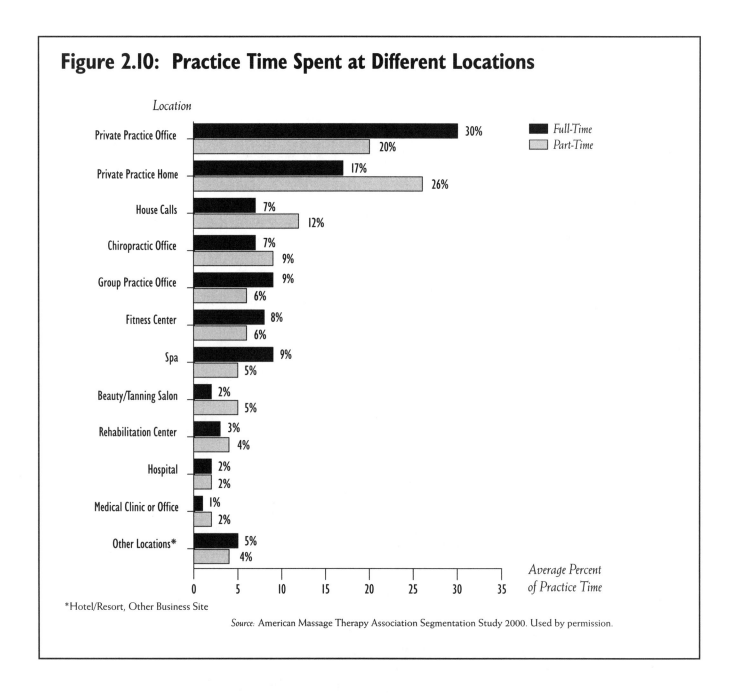

Figure 2.10: Practice Time Spent at Different Locations

Location

Location	Full-Time	Part-Time
Private Practice Office	30%	20%
Private Practice Home	17%	26%
House Calls	7%	12%
Chiropractic Office	7%	9%
Group Practice Office	9%	6%
Fitness Center	8%	6%
Spa	9%	5%
Beauty/Tanning Salon	2%	5%
Rehabilitation Center	3%	4%
Hospital	2%	2%
Medical Clinic or Office	1%	2%
Other Locations*	5%	4%

■ Full-Time
▨ Part-Time

Average Percent of Practice Time

*Hotel/Resort, Other Business Site

Source: American Massage Therapy Association Segmentation Study 2000. Used by permission.

where AMTA members, on average, spend most of their work time.

The Importance of an Office

If you intend to provide all massages on-site, at the locations where your clients live or work, it might seem simplest not to set up any office. Where, then, will you keep business records, make phone calls, and store supplies? If you have a place set aside for these needs, you can be more organized. Also, you may be able to write off the costs of this space against your revenues to lower your income taxes. Thus, you may be better off setting up an office—even one as modest as a small desk in a corner of your home—that you dedicate exclusively to your practice.

Home or Away?

Deciding whether to locate a practice at home or in a separate space combines issues of values and feelings with practical considerations. "Pros and Cons of a Home Office" (figure 2.11, page 70) and "Pros and Cons of a Separate Business Location" (figure 2.12, page 70) summarize the aspects to consider for each type of location. As you review them, consider your own situation, values, and comfort level. For example, some people prefer to practice at home to be near their children. They value having less of a division between their work lives and their family lives. For others, the distinction of maintaining an office separate from their home helps them maintain a professional distance from work. Also, even if you start out at home, eventually you might want to rent office space so that you are better positioned to expand your practice.

An attraction of a home office is the ability to write off some costs related to home ownership (or renting) as business expenses. Ask an accountant for professional advice regarding whether your home office qualifies for deductions. Some possibilities for deductions include:

- A share of the mortgage interest or rent payment (possibly 15 percent if 15 percent of the home's space is devoted solely to the massage therapy practice)
- A share of the property taxes and property insurance (if you deduct a share for business expenses, you may not also deduct the full amount as personal expenses)
- A share of the utilities (electricity, gas, water, garbage collection)
- A share of maintenance costs (for example, repairing the furnace, buying cleaning supplies)
- Phone services devoted to the business (either a separate phone line or the share of the home's phone bill exceeding the basic cost of the phone service and attributable to the business)

Of course, writing off these business expenses, even if and when your accountant advises you that they are qualified, does not make them free. If you are planning on a home-based massage therapy practice, you will need to occupy a home with adequate and appropriate space for the business, and you will have to forego using this space for family activities if you want to claim it as a business expense.

Shared Wisdom

"When setting up a business, don't be shy, be visible. Choose, for example, storefront office space; advertise in the yellow pages, in the newspaper, in alternative newspapers. Participate in health fairs and give demonstrations at your local health food store. Visibility is a great strategy."

—*Chris Hoffman, Finger Lakes Community College, Canandaigua, New York*

Figure 2.11 Pros and Cons of a Home Office

PROS	CONS
Easy to set up, assuming existing home has enough room.	May take space away from family and recreational activities.
Ability to write off portion of home expenses as business expenses.	May require buying or renting a larger home than otherwise needed.
No commuting time (or pollution).	Less separation from work demands at home and from family demands at work.
Possibly the least expensive way to set up a practice.	Safety and security challenges of working alone in a home.
Control over environment, including noise, heat, air, odors.	Clients may feel awkward about coming to your home.
Convenient; close to family.	Americans with Disabilities Act requirements must be met even in a home office.
"Homier" image.	Layout possibly not suitable for business space or for targeted clients (for example, no separate entrance to keep clients from your living area). Potential for conveying less than professional image if you have to lead clients to the "bedroom area" of your home for sessions.

Figure 2.12 Pros and Cons of a Separate Business Location

PROS	CONS
Parking may be more available than in a residential area.	Requires commuting to work (time-consuming and polluting); separation from family.
Helps the massage therapist set boundaries between work and personal.	Less control over the environment, including noise, heat, odors.
Building may already be in compliance with Americans with Disabilities Act requirements and zoned for business.	Requires negotiating a lease and paying rent (which may cost more than for a residence).
Presence of others in an office building a possible asset in terms of safety and security.	Building management may be less concerned about security or noise than you are.
May be more convenient for a massage therapist with a relatively small home.	May require expenses (such as phone line, washer and dryer, computer) for items that you already have at home but are standing idle while you work.

Legal Considerations of Location Selection

In deciding whether to set up your practice at home, you must weigh some legal issues as well. Under the Americans with Disabilities Act, the federal government requires that most businesses serving the public be accessible to people with disabilities. This means that for legal as well as service reasons, you will need to evaluate the accessibility of your home. Can people get in and out easily, even if they use a walker, crutches, or a wheelchair? Where can they use bathroom facilities? Door handles and faucets that are lever-shaped are easier to manipulate than round knobs. Will you have to modify your home for clients?

Many cities and towns have zoning ordinances that specify whether home offices are permitted, or the circumstances under which they are permitted. For example, you might be able to set up a home office if you limit the number of clients who come each week. Or you might be able to do paperwork at home but do all your massage therapy at client sites.

Contact your city's business development or economic development office, or visit the public library and look up your community's zoning ordinances. If you find it difficult to learn whether zoning ordinances affect you, you may want to have an attorney help. Keep in mind that zoning restrictions on home businesses often are stricter than those for businesses in commercial zones. See "Home Office Zoning Regulation Provisions" (figure 2.13, page 72) for possible restrictions.

Local requirements could include:
    bathrooms available
    storage for clean linens
    storage for dirty linens
    lighting requirements
    sink in room
    might have to be affiliated with a doctor or a salon
    might require change in zoning

Be neighborly. Rather than merely learning what the law permits, consider the impact of your practice on your neighbors. If clients will come to your home, where will they park? Will the number of clients affect the traffic or noise level of your neighborhood? Tell your neighbors why people are visiting you several days a week. Such courtesy could pay off for your practice: your neighbors could become your clients. [Source: Sohnen-Moe, Cherie. "Zoning: Your Rights and Responsibilities." *Massage Therapy Journal*, Spring 1999, pages 70-71, 74, 76.]

Safety Considerations

Operating a home office also introduces certain safety considerations if you will see clients there. In particular, you and the client(s) may be the only ones in the building at some times. You must be prepared to handle all your own emergencies as well as inappropriate client behavior. For more information on safety and security issues, see "Safety and Security Precautions" in chapter 4, pages 180-181.

Figure 2.13

If you need to file with your municipality for a home-office zoning variance, check your local zoning ordinances to find out what is required. The following descriptions might be helpful in making your case.

❑ The home office or business is clearly secondary to the use of the dwelling as a residence and does not change the residential character of the dwelling or the lot in any visible manner.

❑ The work done in the home office or business creates no objectionable odor, noticeable vibration, or offensive noise that increases the level of ambient sound at the property lines.

❑ The home office or business does not cause unsightly conditions or waste visible off the property.

❑ The home office or business does not cause interference with radio or television reception in the vicinity.

❑ The home office or business has no more than two full-time employees who are not residents of the household. Special permits may be granted to allow more employees.

❑ The home office or business has no signs visible from the street that are inconsistent with signs allowed elsewhere in the zoning regulations.

❑ The home office or business sells no articles at retail on the premises that are not made or grown on the premises.

❑ The home office or business occupies less than half the floor areas of the dwelling.

❑ The home office or business has sufficient off-street parking for both the residential and the business uses of the dwelling.

❑ The home office or business does not create a volume of passenger or commercial traffic that is inconsistent with the normal level of traffic on the street on which the dwelling is located.

Source: Kiné-Concept Institute Business Success Workbook, as adapted from a model ordinance developed by the National Alliance of Home Businesswomen, an organization that supports the working-from-home movement.

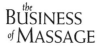

© 2002 American Massage Therapy Association, Evanston, IL. *The Business of Massage.* All Rights Reserved. #20026

Buying an Existing Practice vs. Creating One

A massage therapy practice may feel more like a way of life than a business, but in fact it is also a collection of assets and liabilities that can be bought and sold. Because buying any kind of business is a sophisticated transaction, be sure to get qualified legal and financial advice before you consider buying a massage therapy practice.

Why might you decide to buy a massage therapy practice, rather than starting your own? There are a few possible reasons:

- You may be able to earn a profit faster if the practice is already established.
- You would start out using a practice name that has already acquired a good reputation and client base. However, if one massage therapist sells a practice to another, it is important for the therapist making the purchase to consider whether clients will see it as the same practice, or just someone else operating under the same name. In other words, you might pay extra for an established practice, only to lose most of the clients after the purchase is complete.
- A "package deal" may be simpler than hunting for each item needed to set up an office. However, make sure that among the benefits you enjoy is an ongoing client base. Otherwise, it might be cheaper to offer to buy the used massage tables and some equipment, rather than the practice itself. Also, be sure before you buy that each element of the practice meets your standards for quality.

If you decide to purchase a massage therapy practice, you must consider all the issues that arise when you start a practice. Find out why the practice owner wants to sell. Consider the office space and where it is located. Go over all the business records with your attorney. Examine all the financial records with your accountant, asking questions about anything you do not understand. Finally, before you buy, get answers to the following questions:

- Does the practice generate enough earnings every month to meet your financial goals?
- How many one-hour massage sessions does the practice provide each month? How many are to repeat customers?
- Has the practice been operating according to all the applicable laws and regulations?
- Will you be committed to the lease agreement that is already in place? If so, for how long?
- If you had set up the office yourself, would you have done it the same way?
- Will making changes be harder or more costly than setting it up your way in the first place?
- Are the practice's standards, goals, and philosophy compatible with your own?
- If there are employees, are they planning on staying?

In "How Much Is Your Business Worth?" author Lloyd R. Manning recommends that a massage therapy business owner use the following criteria in valuing his or her practice:

- Fees charged and maintainable
- Past, present, and anticipated level of earnings
- Length of time the practice has been established
- Reputation of the practice

Shared Wisdom

"If you want to buy an existing practice, consider the option of renting to own. You might agree with the owner that you will run the practice for one year and give the owner 80% of your fees, which accrue to the purchase. At the end of the year, you own the business. Or, if you have decided at the end of the year that you don't want the business, the owner keeps what you have already paid in. The agreement should be in writing. This provides subsistence living for you (the buyer) the first year, but it allows for gradual payment and the smooth and gradual transition from the first owner."

—Barry Antoniow, Kiné-Concept Institute - Maritimes, Fredericton, New Brunswick, Canada

- Location considerations, occupancy cost, and remaining lease term
- Types and affluence of the clients
- Level of competition
- Ease of starting a new practice
- Number of persons seeking this type of practice, in this locale

Source: Lloyd R. Manning. "How Much Is Your Business Worth?" *Massage Therapy Journal*, Spring 2001, pages 102-110.

If your examination of the practice still supports your belief that purchasing it is a good move, determine whether you have the necessary funding to complete the purchase. Will you have enough left to live on until you can begin collecting revenue from the practice? It is probably wise to assume that some faithful clients will stop coming when ownership changes hands, but you should also be ready to identify sources of new clients. Also, be sure the sales agreement includes a non-compete clause, in case the owner later wants to continue practicing in the area. Finally, be sure to follow the same good business practices as you would if you were setting up a new practice.

Equipment and Supplies

What equipment and supplies will you need to outfit your business? Chapter 4 contains details regarding the selection of equipment and supplies that fit the image and service of your business. See "Equipping Your Massage Therapy Practice" (figure 4.13, page 184) for a list of furniture, equipment, and supplies. Chapter 4 also contains information about compliance with the Americans with Disabilities Act, which could influence your furniture and equipment purchase decisions.

Hiring Employees

You might decide, even when you first open your practice, that you want to work with others, in either an employer/employee or a client/independent contractor relationship. Information regarding the hiring process is contained in this section. More information regarding supervising and managing employees is covered in chapter 3.

Hiring employees improves the capacity of your practice to serve clients. It also greatly increases your responsibilities as a business owner. Therefore, before you take that step, review "Pros and Cons of Hiring an Employee" (figure 2.14, page 75). Then answer these questions:
- Am I thinking about hiring someone because I know, or anticipate, that I cannot complete the workload myself? If so, do I want to manage a larger practice? Would I be more satisfied if I consider other ways to keep up with my workload (such as reducing the number of clients I serve or contracting with an accountant to do my taxes)?
- Am I thinking about hiring someone because I don't want to work alone? If so, would I be more satisfied with a partner, or with becoming an employee myself?
- Would I obtain the same benefits more easily by subleasing space (if my lease permits), charging therapists a share of the rent or a percentage of their fees?

- Am I thinking about hiring someone because I would like to focus on the administrative and marketing aspects of the practice and let someone else handle the massage sessions? If so, do I have the necessary skills?
- Will I have enough work for the person I hire to do year-round? Or am I anticipating being too busy during just a peak period that will later level off?

It is crucial to be clear about your decision to hire someone. That person will depend on you for a livelihood. You may want to start with a trial period to decide whether you and the employee are compatible. Otherwise, if you decide a few months later that you cannot afford or do not really want this person to work for you, your hiring decision was ultimately harmful to the employee.

Despite the complexity and expense of hiring employees, they can be valuable assets of your practice. When you hire the right people, you establish ongoing ties with them and have the right to expect them to meet your guidelines. Entering into an independent contractor arrangement is simpler in some ways. However, you have less control over what the contractor does. The employment agreement (figure 2.15, page 76) and independent contractor agreement samples (figure 2.19, page 82) illustrate the issues to consider when setting up both types of arrangements.

Figure 2.14: Pros and Cons of Hiring an Employee

PROS	CONS
More people can get more work done.	You must spend time training and supervising each employee.
A qualified employee can be expected to follow your work systems and policies.	You must learn and comply with a host of labor and tax laws.
An employee can expand the range of skills and talents available in your practice.	You must have a consistent source of funds to pay your employee (and the withholding taxes).
A greater number of people can increase scheduling flexibility.	Your practice could be liable for harm done by an employee in the course of his or her employment.
Another person can build teamwork and make you feel less isolated.	You must cover for an ill employee, which can require double work or rescheduling clients.
	You might have to address issues related to absenteeism or unsatisfactory performance.

Figure 2.15

This Agreement is hereby made this_____day of _____, _____ between

(date)   (month)   (year)

_____, located at _____ ("Employer")

(name of massage therapy clinic/business)   (street address, city, state, ZIP—can be therapist's residence)

and_____, residing at _____ ("Employee")

(name of massage therapist)   (street address, city, state, ZIP)

for the performance of massage therapy services according to the following terms and conditions:

I. Tasks to Be Performed, Equipment, and Supplies

1.1   In the course of his/her employment, Employee shall primarily be required to perform massage therapy. However, when not engaged in treatments, Employee shall be required to assist other practitioners with clients, perform clerical duties when requested, and participate in the cleaning and organizing of Employer's place of business.

1.2   Employee shall provide massage therapy services only within the limits and scope of his/her knowledge and/or licensure, if applicable, and is responsible for maintaining appropriate certification and licensure (including all costs thereof unless otherwise agreed).

1.3   Employee shall dress in a style consistent with Employer's image, including uniforms the purchase of which may or may not be the responsibility of Employee.

1.4   Employee shall maintain client records in the manner prescribed by Employer, the same to be and remain the property of Employer.

1.5   Employer shall supply, at its sole expense, all equipment, tools, materials, and/or supplies necessary for Employee to perform the tasks set forth in this Section 1, including but not limited to (list all equipment, etc. that will be supplied, i.e., room, table, draping, oils, lotions, music, marketing materials, etc.).

1.6   Employee shall be required to work_____hours per week according to a schedule set forth by Employer.

2. Compensation

2.1   Employer shall pay Employee twice monthly at a rate of $_____per hour worked plus an additional $_____per half hour massage performed and $_____per one hour massage performed.

2.2   Employer shall be responsible for paying all required federal, state, and local withholding, social security and Medicare taxes.

2.3   Employee may participate in any Employer benefit program as Employee becomes eligible.

2.4   Employer shall provide/maintain insurance coverage for workers' compensation, unemployment, general liability, fire, and theft.

the
BUSINESS
of MASSAGE

© 2002 American Massage Therapy Association, Evanston, IL. *The Business of Massage.* All Rights Reserved. #20026

3. Term And Termination

3.1 This Employment Agreement is effective as of the date first written above and shall continue in effect until terminated by either party, given reasonable cause, or upon thirty (30) days written notice to the other party of the intention to terminate.

3.2 The following are considered reasonable cause:

    a. Failure of either party to perform the obligations under the Agreement;

    b. Action by either party exposing the other to liability for property damage or personal injury;

    c. Violation of applicable ethical standards and/or loss of licensure for services provided;

    d. Failure of Employee to maintain the standard of service deemed appropriate by Employer; or

    e. Employee's engagement in any pattern or course of conduct on a continuing basis which adversely affects Employee's, Employer's, or other employees' ability to perform services.

3.3 Termination of this Agreement shall not relieve Employer of its obligation to pay Employee any monies due and owing even if such monies are not due until after the date of termination.

4. Additional Provisions

4.1 Employee has the right to perform similar services for others during the term of this Agreement, however, such services may not be performed on Employer's premises.

4.2 During the term of this Agreement and for six (6) months after termination, Employee shall not solicit Employer's clients or employees for private practice.

4.3 Any of the Employee's independent marketing materials must be approved in advance prior to their display or distribution to Employer's clients.

4.4 The provisions of this Agreement shall be interpreted and enforced in accordance with the laws of the State of_____. All unresolved disputes arising out of this Agreement shall be finally settled by Arbitration.

4.5 This document represents the entire agreement of the parties with regard to the employment of Employee and supersedes any and all prior written or verbal agreements. Any amendments to this Agreement must be in writing and signed by both parties. Should any provisions of this Agreement be deemed unenforceable, the remainder of the Agreement shall continue in effect.

_____   _____
Employer Signature   Employee Signature

_____   _____
Employer Name   Employee Name

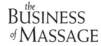

the
BUSINESS
of MASSAGE

© 2002 American Massage Therapy Association, Evanston, IL. *The Business of Massage.* All Rights Reserved. #20026

If you determine that you want to hire an employee, you must begin advertising the position and selecting candidates. Ask for leads from people who might know someone with the desired background. You can also look in job banks and place advertisements in local and trade publications. Many people advise against hiring friends and family.

Decide ahead of time qualifications that are important to you. How will you measure those qualifications in an employee? Will you need advice from a mentor or someone else with experience in making employment decisions? Be sure to check the references provided by each applicant, especially when hiring someone who will work with your money or your clients.

Several important laws affect how you will go about the process of screening candidates and selecting an employee. To avoid costly lawsuits, be sure to learn what you can and cannot ask. Some of the laws to become familiar with are as follows:

- Antidiscrimination laws such as the Civil Rights Act prohibit you from selecting employees on the basis of race, color, religion, sex, national origin, age (for adults under age 70), or marital status.
- The Americans with Disabilities Act (ADA), passed by Congress in 1990, forbids discrimination based on disability (assuming the person can do the essential tasks of the job). It requires that employers make reasonable accommodations to permit disabled employees to do their work. (It also requires that businesses serving the public make their facilities accessible to people with disabilities.)
- The Federal Immigration Reform and Control Act of 1986 requires that employers verify that they hire only people who are eligible to work in the United States. However, it also prohibits employers from discriminating against eligible foreign workers.

To help you comply with these laws, "Sample Questions for Employers to Ask and to Avoid During an Employment Interview" (figure 2.16, below) gives a few examples of questions to ask and questions to avoid during an employment interview. Be sure you are fully knowledgeable about what is and isn't acceptable to ask.

Figure 2.16 Sample Questions for Employers to Ask and to Avoid During an Employment Interview

Questions to Ask	Questions to Avoid
What have you learned during your experience as a massage therapist?	How old are you? What is your religion?
Our office is open on evenings and weekends. Will you be able to work those hours? (To learn whether a person will be available on evenings and weekends)	Do you have little children? (To learn whether a person will be available on evenings and weekends)
Some of the potential clients in our area speak Spanish, Portuguese, and possibly other languages. What languages do you speak fluently?	What country are you from? What kind of an accent do you have?

Complying with Employment Laws

Many employers do not understand all of the employment laws. Fortunately, common sense and fairness go a long way toward preventing problems.

- To comply with antidiscrimination laws, be very specific about the qualifications for which you are looking. Think in terms of abilities, education, and experience. When you interview candidates, focus on those qualities, rather than other attributes that may not be relevant. For example, wrongfully assuming that the gender, age, or race of a potential employee will make clients uncomfortable is discriminatory. Further, it prevents you from seriously considering candidates who may be well qualified and skilled in client relations.
- The same advice holds for complying with ADA. Focus on qualifications. If you wonder how a person with a disability could perform a particular task, you can ask the applicant to perform it so you can see if he or she is able to accomplish the task. You might have to make some accommodations, but if you have made your practice accessible to clients already, chances are it will be accessible to most employees.
- To comply with the Immigration Reform and Control Act, you must be sure everyone you hire provides proof of citizenship or authorization to work in the United States. Have each person complete Form I-9, Employment Eligibility Verification, available from the U.S. Immigration and Naturalization Service. The INS also publishes an information handbook titled Handbook for Employers: Instructions for Completing Form I-9. To ensure compliance or to get answers to any questions about these laws, obtain advice from an attorney familiar with employment matters.

Complying with these employment laws can prevent costly lawsuits.

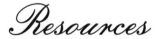

Where to Find Massage Therapists to Hire
- placement offices and job postings at schools provide relevant training referrals from friends and colleagues
- placing want ads in local newspapers
- ads for massage therapists in the AMTA Job Network: www.amtamassage.org
- independent Web sites that allow posting of jobs, such as: www.healingartsresource.com
- want ads in professional journals (e.g., *Massage Therapy Journal* and *Massage Magazine*)

Work Hours and Scheduling

Your business planning worksheet should describe anyone who will work with or for you, as well as the number of hours you want to work, or the number of sessions you want per week. For a basis of comparison, about half of AMTA members work full-time as massage therapists. "Number of Paid Hours Per Week" (figure 2.17, below) shows the number of paid sessions per week provided by AMTA members.

Figure 2.17 Number of Paid Hours Per Week

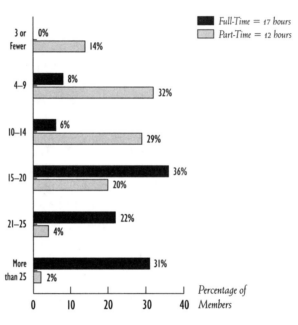

Number of Paid Massage Hours/Week

■ Full-Time = 17 hours
▨ Part-Time = 12 hours

Percentage of Members

AMTA generally describes full-time as more than 17 hours a week, and part-time as less than 17 hours a week. Responses to this survey, however, indicate that some practitioners who give fewer than 17 hours of massage per week consider themselves full-time, and some who give more than 17 hours consider themselves part-time.

Source: American Massage Therapy Association Segmentation Study 2000. Used by permission.

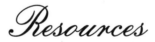

Information Regarding Employment Laws
- Equal Employment Opportunity Commission (1-800-669-4000 or www.eeoc.gov)—information about antidiscrimination laws and Americans with Disabilities Act
- Immigration and Naturalization Service (www.ins.usdoj.gov), or get the phone number for your local office from the government pages of your phone book)
- Information about the Immigration Reform and Control Act

Using Independent Contractors

Given the many requirements involved with hiring employees, many massage therapists prefer to get help in the form of independent contractors. An independent contractor provides a service, but not as an employee. From the employer's perspective, the main differences are summarized in "Employee versus Independent Contractor: The Employer's Perspective" (figure 2.18, below). To avoid the obligations of an employer by contracting with people instead of hiring them, be sure to treat them as independent. In other words, you cannot tell independent contractors how to go about the work they do for you—what steps to follow, what hours to be in the office, and so on. Instead, you must agree on the end result of the work, then select people you trust to do the job in an acceptable way.

An independent contractor will charge a fee that amounts to more earnings per hour than an employee would receive. After all, independent contractors need to earn enough to provide their own benefits, such as insurance, time off from work, and so on. On the other hand, you are paying independent contractors only for the specific tasks contracted for (not for the occasional slow week), so you may still come out ahead.

Figure 2.18: Employee versus Independent Contractor: The Employer's Perspective

Employee	*Independent Contractor*
Can be instructed to follow specific rules and procedures	Must be free to determine how and when to complete a project
An ongoing work relationship	Relationship limited to scope of project(s) contracted for
Paid a wage or salary, with taxes withheld	Paid a fee, with no taxes withheld
Share of social security taxes paid by employer	Responsible for paying self-employment tax
May expect benefits in addition to pay (standard value is about 15 percent of pay)	Expects a fee large enough to provide self with benefits
Employment relationship covered by antidiscrimination and labor laws	Contracting relationship covered by contract law
May not be available at times needed	

Figure 2.19

This Agreement is hereby made this_____day of _____ , _____between
                                         (date)   (month)   (year)
_____ , a provider of massage therapy services with its principal office
(name of massage therapist/massage therapy business)
located at _____("Independent Contractor") and
              (street address, city, state, ZIP—can be therapist's residence)
_____ , with its principal place of business at _____ ("Client"),
(name of clinic/business/hirer of services)   (street address, city, state, ZIP)
for massage therapy services at Client's place of business according to the following terms and conditions:

I. Services To Be Provided, Equipment And Supplies

1.1   Independent Contractor agrees to provide Massage Therapy Services ("Services") at Client's place of business to patrons of Client within the limits and scope of its knowledge and/or licensure, if applicable. (A specific description of the massage therapy services that will be made available can be included.)

1.2   Independent Contractor shall supply, at its sole expense, all equipment, tools, materials, and/or supplies necessary to provide the Services except for the following: (List any equipment, etc. provided by Client, e.g., massage table or chair, towel cart, room with sink and countertop, appointment scheduling for Client's patrons, insurance billing).

1.3   Independent Contractor shall set his/her own hours, but agrees to be available to patrons of Client a minimum of _____hours per week. For scheduling purposes, Independent Contractor shall attempt to be available on a consistent basis, and agrees to notify Client if his/her availability will change.

2. Fees And Terms Of Payment

2.1   Independent Contractor shall set the fee charged to patrons of Client for Services.

2.2   Client shall collect said fees on behalf of Independent Contractor and shall remit the same to Independent Contractor, less 30% to cover operating expenses, room rental, and equipment usage, within five (5) days of receipt.

2.3   No federal, state, or local income tax or payroll tax of any kind shall be withheld or paid by Client on behalf of Independent Contractor. Independent Contractor shall be solely responsible for all tax liability.

3. Expense Reimbursement, Fringe Benefits, Insurance

3.1   Client shall not be liable to Independent Contractor for any expenses paid or incurred by Independent Contractor unless otherwise agreed to in writing.

3.2   Independent Contractor acknowledges that because it is not an employee of Client, it is not eligible for and shall not participate in any employer benefits of the Client, including pension, health, or other fringe benefits.

3.3   No worker's compensation or unemployment insurance shall be obtained by Client concerning Independent Contractor or employees thereof. Independent Contractor agrees to comply with all workers' compensation laws concerning its business, and if a corporation, shall provide Client a certificate of workers' compensation insurance.

3.4   Independent Contractor shall furnish Client with current certificates of coverage and proof of payment for all applicable insurance, including, but not limited to liability insurance with minimum coverage of $_____aggregate annual and $_____per occurrence.

the
BUSINESS
of MASSAGE

© 2002 American Massage Therapy Association, Evanston, IL. *The Business of Massage.* All Rights Reserved. #20026

4. Term And Termination

4.1   This Contract for Massage Therapy Services is effective as of the date first written above and shall continue in effect until terminated by either party upon thirty (30) days written notice to the other party.

4.2   Termination of this Contract shall not relieve Client of its obligation to pay Independent Contractor any monies due and owing even if such monies are not due until after the date of termination.

4.3   This notice required by this Section shall be sent to the respective addresses set forth above via (I) certified mail, return receipt requested, (II) overnight or second-day courier delivery, or (III) facsimile message if a confirmation copy is sent by one of the methods set forth in subsection (I) or (II). Notice shall be deemed given when received by the other party.

4.4   During the term of this Contract and for six months after termination, Independent Contractor shall not solicit patrons or employees for any purposes.

5. Additional Provisions

5.1   By Independent Contractor. Independent Contractor agrees and acknowledges:

a.   that it will dress in a style consistent with the Client's image;

b.   that it will maintain patron records in a mutually agreed manner;

c.   that all patron records remain the property of Client unless otherwise agreed;

d.   that it has no authority to enter into contracts or agreements on behalf of Client;

e.   that it has complied with all applicable laws regarding business permits, certificates, and/or licenses that may be required to carry out the Services to be performed under this Contract;

f.   that it will indemnify and hold Client harmless from any and all loss or liability arising out of or incurred as a result of the performance of Services under this Contract.

5.2   By Client. Client agrees and acknowledges:

a.   that Independent Contractor may perform similar services for others during the term of this Contract;

b.   that it has no control over the means, manners, and method by which the Services are provided;

c.   that it has no authority to enter into contracts or agreements on behalf of Independent Contractor.

5.3   Assignment. This Contract may not be assigned, in whole or in part, by either party without the express written consent of the other party.

5.4   Choice of Law. Any dispute under this Contract or related to this Contract shall be decided in accordance with the laws of the State of_____.

5.5   Entire Agreement. This document represents the entire agreement of the parties with regard to the provision of Services and supersedes any and all prior written or verbal agreements. Any amendments to this Contract must be in writing and signed by both parties. Should any provision of this Contract be deemed unenforceable, the remainder of the Contract shall continue in effect.

_____
Independent Contractor Signature

_____
Client Signature

_____
Independent Contractor Name

_____
Client Name

the
BUSINESS
of MASSAGE

© 2002 American Massage Therapy Association, Evanston, IL. *The Business of Massage.* All Rights Reserved. #20026

Communications Strategies for Negotiating an Independent Contractor Agreement

Whether you intend to become an independent contractor or you hire one, the issues surrounding negotiating a contract concern fair treatment of both the person who is contracted and the business that does the contracting. Both parties need to feel confident that the business arrangement will lead to mutual value and a good working relationship with each other and with your mutual clients. As you enter into contract negotiations from either side of the negotiating table, you will want to discuss the following areas:

Services, Equipment and Supplies
- Will the independent contractor provide his or her massage table, linens, oils and lotions?
- Who pays for laundry?
- How much flexibility will the independent contractor have in furnishing/decorating the session room?
- What does the business offer in terms of privacy for clients, control of heat/air in the session room, rest room proximity, and other amenities?
- Will the receptionist at the business make appointments for the independent contractor? Who pays the receptionist?
- Will the independent contractor work during set hours, or only by appointment? If only by appointment, will the session room be available at all times?
- Does the independent contractor set his or her own policies regarding cancellation, tipping, appropriate dress, etc.?
- Does the independent contractor have the authority to subcontract to another practitioner and allow that person to use the same space?

Fees and Terms of Payment
- Who sets the independent contractors' fees?
- Who collects payment from clients?
- Will the business do any advertising or marketing of the independent contractor's services?
- Who pays for business cards that show the business contact information?
- Will the independent contractor rent space from the business?
- Will the independent contractor pay the business a percentage of fees from massage sessions?
- Will the business guarantee a minimum number of clients or fees to the independent contractor per month?
- Does the independent contractor or the business have the ability to set a maximum number of appointments per week or month?
- Is the fee percentage split based on a specified number of massage appointments per week or month?
- Does the fee percentage split stay the same regardless of the number of appointments?
- If the independent contractor brings in his or her own clients, is the fee percentage split the same as when the business generates the appointment?

Expense Reimbursement and Insurance
- Are there any expenses of the independent contractor for which the business will be responsible?
- What documentation does the business require that shows the independent contractor's paid liability insurance coverage?

Additional Provisions
- Who owns client records?
- What credentials does the business require that show the level of training of the independent contractor?

Terms and Termination
- What is the duration of the independent contractor agreement?
- What are the terms for ending the agreement prior to its expiration date?

Your Financial Objectives and Plans

Be as specific as you can about your financial objectives and plans. You need to be sure you can afford your plans. Completing all the information in this section of the "Career and Practice Planning Worksheet" (at end of this chapter) can help you decide whether you need to modify your plans in order to be profitable.

To complete the financial section of your career planning worksheet, you will need to estimate your start-up costs, your monthly expenses, and your revenues. This is similar to when you estimated supply and demand of your client base and the number of available massage therapists in your area, but this adds in the financial overhead not included in the supply and demand model. These are the categories to plan for:

Start-Up Costs
- printing business cards, stationery, brochures
- dues for professional association membership and other business organizations, such as chamber of commerce
- correspondence with professionals and other networking contacts
- cost of setting up office and/or practice space in home or other location
- rent (and initial deposit) for office/practice space
- purchase of equipment and supplies
- fees for professional services, such as attorney, accountant
- government fees, such as license, business license tax, or incorporation fees
- liability insurance
- other costs

Estimating Monthly Expenses
When you create your business plan, make an estimate of your monthly expenses. These expenses are likely to fall into the following categories, as shown on the "Career and Practice Planning Worksheet":
- marketing communication pieces, such as brochures, signs, and ads
- rent/mortgage payments for your work space
- supplies
- merchandise to sell
- loan payments
- phone and utilities

- employees' pay
- professional services, such as attorney and accountant
- taxes (property, business, income)
- insurance (liability, disability, health)
- membership fees
- continuing education
- professional publications
- other expenses, such as equipment, school loans, and laundry

Estimating Monthly Revenues

Your revenues are likely to fall into three primary categories:
- revenue from massage sessions
- revenue from product sales
- fees from associate who shares space with you (if any)

Your Breakeven Analysis

When you estimate your revenues and expenses, you may be surprised at how long it will take you to break even. See "Breakeven Analysis" (figure 2.20, page 87) for an example of how to calculate whether your monthly expenses and revenue will allow you to break even. If your first estimate shows that your expenses will be higher than your revenue, see if you can adjust your estimates by planning to work a few more hours each month or reducing your expenses, while still staying within a realistic framework.

When you are satisfied with your estimates, convert the estimated revenue into the number of clients you will need to meet your calendar for breaking even:

Estimated monthly revenue

Divided by your hourly fee

Equals number of massage hours per month

As you complete your breakeven analysis and review the other ideas in this section, you may realize that you need another source of funding to pay your bills as you get started. Some people are fortunate enough to have a spouse, family member, or other person who will provide for their financial needs while they work toward financial stability.

If you need some other source of funding, can you take on a full- or part-time job to cover expenses while getting started as a massage therapist? (Be sure the job leaves you with enough energy to do your best as a therapist.) Other ways to get funding are to borrow from a bank or credit union, or to form a partnership with someone who has the money to invest. If you are starting out on your own, your credit cards are an easy source of funds. But be careful! It is easy to run up big bills at a high interest rate without really thinking through how to make the monthly payments that must follow soon after.

Figure 2.20

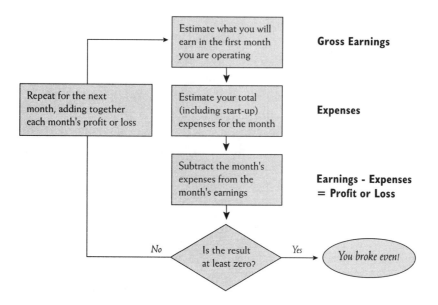

When you estimate your revenues and expenses, you may be surprised at how long it will take you to break even. To continue your breakeven analysis, adjust your estimates. For example, to break even sooner, try working a few more hours each month. Estimate the change in monthly revenues and expenses. Now redo the breakeven analysis with your new numbers.

When you are satisfied with your estimates, convert the estimated revenue into the number of clients you will need to meet your calendar for breaking even:

Estimated monthly revenue	$ _____
Divided by your hourly fee	÷ _____
Equals number of massage hours per month	= _____
Divided by number of massage hours for an average client in a month	÷ _____
Equals number of clients per month to achieve estimated revenue	= _____

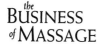

© 2002 American Massage Therapy Association, Evanston, IL. *The Business of Massage*. All Rights Reserved. #20026

Applying for Funds

If you want to get funding, whether by borrowing from a bank or by sharing ownership (as in a partnership or corporation), you will need to present your plans in an organized way. People who invest in your practice will want some assurance that you will use their money wisely. One way to demonstrate this is to prepare a business plan. To do so, use the information in the "Career and Practice Planning Worksheet" to write a plan with the following categories:

- *Summary*—your goals
- *Background*—description of the demand already met by other massage therapy practitioners in your area, the additional community needs you have identified, and your qualifications to meet those needs
- *Marketing*—your target market (the categories of clients you plan to serve), the services and products you plan to offer, their prices, and the ways you will use marketing communications in your practice
- *Operations*—where you will practice, what equipment you will use, who you will work with, how you will provide for adequate staffing and training
- *Financing*—your needs for start-up funding and where you plan to get the funds; your projected monthly revenues and expenses, including the expense of paying off any loans; the value of your practice's assets (such as equipment you have already obtained for the practice) and liabilities (any money you owe).
- *Conclusion*—how your plans will enable you to meet your financial objectives
- *Attach relevant documents*—Depending on your circumstances, these might include résumés of key people (including yourself), letters of recommendation, tax returns for the past three years, proof of liability insurance, and brochures or other marketing literature for your practice.

Planning for Your Retirement

When you are twenty or thirty years old, retirement seems very far away. And if you are setting up a practice, there are many expenses. However, the sooner you start putting some money into an IRA or other investment, the better off you will be. In Canada, the IRA-equivalent is the Registered Retirement Savings Plan, or RRSP. Compound interest makes the value of your investment rise faster over time. If you save for forty years instead of for twenty, you save for twice as long but earn far more than twice as much. Thus, the sooner you start saving, the more you can benefit from this "magic" of compound interest.

The financial protection that comes from careful recordkeeping can also result from planning for retirement. Someday you will probably want to rest from your successful career. Therefore, you will need to attend to the financial needs of retirement. The specific approaches available to you will depend somewhat on whether you are an employee or operate a business (including a sole proprietorship). Keep in mind that if you have employees but provide retirement benefits only to yourself, you probably will not be able to deduct the cost of these benefits from your business profit.

Most people try to balance risk with return by using more than one method of saving for retirement. A financial adviser can be very helpful when you are making these decisions.

By beginning now to plan for retirement, you will have a nest egg and be able to enjoy what you do even more. Each month, set aside money for taxes and for retirement savings. In later years you will reap the benefits and be glad you prepared. For this reason, it is a good habit to start your retirement plan when you start your practice. Refer to "The Power of Compound Interest" (figure 2.21, below) for a chart that shows how compound interest makes your money work for you. See the resources list, "Sources of Information about Saving for Retirement," for more assistance in this area.

Figure 2.21 The Power of Compound Interest

At an interest rate of	Your investment will double in:
3%	24.0 years
5%	14.4 years
7%	10.3 years
10%	7.2 years
12%	6.0 years
15%	4.8 years
20%	3.6 years

Source: AARP Web site: www.aarp.org/confacts/money/compinterest.html

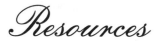

Sources of Information About Saving for Retirement

- your accountant
- your insurance agent (may get a commission for selling you something)
- a Certified Financial Planner (typically will charge a fee for advice, but will not get commissions for selling you something)
- your employer's (or spouse's employer's) human resources department
- Orman, Suze. *The Courage to Be Rich: Creating a Life of Spiritual and Material Abundance* (New York: Riverhead Press, 1999)
- Orman, Suze. *The 9 Steps to Financial Freedom: Practical and Spiritual Steps So You Can Stop Worrying.* New York: Crown Books, 1998.
- Web site for Quicken financial software (www.quicken.com)

Evaluation of Your Plan

In the final section of the "Career and Practice Planning Worksheet," evaluate your plan. Do your ideas support the basic goals you recorded at the beginning of the worksheet? If not, change either your career objectives or the details of your plan. It is better to make changes in the planning stage than to waste precious time, money, and energy on a plan that doesn't hold together solidly from the outset.

Taxes, Contracts, and Other Legal Considerations

Licenses and Permits

Before you accept your first client, make sure you have obtained all the necessary licenses and permits. State and local requirements vary, and you are responsible for finding out what you need. As you gather information, you may discover other requirements for starting your practice, such as zoning regulations. Check with your state departments of revenue and consumer affairs, county clerk, and city hall about the following:

- State, county, and/or city massage therapist license
- City and/or county business license
- City and/or county certificate of occupancy for an office
- State and/or county DBA (for "doing business as") permit for operating your practice under a name other than your own
- Building permits for building or remodeling space
- Permits from your local fire, health, or police department
- Seller's permit for your state, city, or county (if you must charge a sales tax for selling products)
- Employer Identification Number from the IRS (if you are a partnership or corporation or if you hire employees)

License and Permit Fees

Some local governments charge a tax or fee for operating a business. The fee may vary according to the type of business and where it is located. Here are some examples of annual fees and one-time start-up business license fees owed by massage therapists in several locations.

City	Fees
Alaska	$100 for two years (all businesses register through the state; Anchorage also requires a separate city license)
Alberta, Alberta, Canada	$75 annual fee (for a resident of Alberta)

Shared Wisdom

"Don't wait until after graduation to begin looking at the reality of finding work as a professional. Find out the costs of oil and business cards, call three publications and obtain the costs of advertising, provide the name, address, and contact person of three establishments where you might get a job as a massage therapist."

—Sue Brown, Illinois School of Health Careers, Chicago, Illinois

Boulder, Colorado	$25 one-time application fee
Cambridge, Massachusetts	$15 every four years (called a business certificate)
Chicago, Illinois	$250 to operate the business; $125 per individual who provides massage
Fairfield, Virginia	Percentage of gross receipts
Kirksville, Missouri	$25 annual fee ($10 one-time processing fee for first year)
Nashville, Tennessee	$20 annual county fee; $20 annual city fee
Phoenix, Arizona	$295 application fee; $30 annual fee
Santa Cruz, California	$145.15 annual fee, plus $7.40 per employee
Seattle, Washington	$75 annual license fee, plus $10 per branch

Again, it is essential that you contact your own city, county, and state governments to learn whether you will be subject to some form of business tax. To find the requirements of your own city, contact your local government office that handles business services. You might find it listed under such names as city clerk, tax and licensing division, or business license division.

Fees for business licenses and permits are not the same as fees charged by your state for a massage therapy license, which is a professional license. For instance, in Wisconsin, the Title Protection Act says you can't call yourself a massage therapist until: you are licensed, you become state registered, or become nationally certified. Being licensed by the National Certification for Therapeutic Massage and Bodywork (NCTMB) or AOBTA, or registered, demonstrates to the state that you carry $1 million liability insurance, that you graduated from a state-approved school, and that you have not committed a crime. You are also then classified as a healthcare provider, which means you may participate in third-party reimbursement for insurance claims if you choose to.

Property Taxes

If you own the property on which your practice is located, you may have to pay a state property tax. If you operate out of your home, and if you own (rather than rent) your home, the portion of property taxes you attribute to your home office would be considered an expense of your practice. For example, suppose you have set up an office that you use exclusively for your practice, and it occupies one-fifth of the square footage of your home. Usually you then can deduct one-fifth of your property taxes as a business expense; however, be sure that you do not also deduct that portion as a personal expense on your personal tax return. It is best to consult an accountant about a property tax deduction such as this.

Insurance—Protecting Yourself from Loss

Along with other key business concerns such as retirement planning, setting up an office, and preparing marketing materials, you should plan to use insurance to protect yourself from work time losses such as being hospitalized or losing your home in a fire. When you set up a massage therapy practice, your coverage needs increase. The types of insurance are described below:

1. *Professional liability (also known as malpractice or personal injury) insurance*

   This coverage protects you against claims by clients that they were injured because of the work you did. It is essential for every massage therapist, and is included in most memberships to professional associations. Professional liability insurance protects the policyholder from wrongful advice or errors on the practitioner's behalf, which allegedly lead to some kind of harm to the client. It also covers claims that are related to the "scope of practice," that is, the services you provide in your capacity as a professional massage therapist.

   Professional liability rates are affordable in the massage therapy profession, largely because there haven't been many claims against your peers in the profession. This absence of claims is to some degree attributable to the ethical standards massage therapists follow, and the care with which services are rendered. In order to maintain the excellent record in the profession, practitioners must abide by these guidelines:
   - Do not use terms that imply that you are offering diagnoses for ailments, or treatment that addresses any ailment. Massage therapists do not have the authority to prescribe medical solutions, diagnose conditions, or offer specific treatment for cures.
   - Get a second opinion from a physician if the client complains of symptoms that may suggest contraindications for massage.

2. *General liability ("slip and fall") insurance*

   This coverage protects you against claims that a person or his or her property was injured on your property or because of something you did outside your capacity as a professional (for example, spilling coffee on a client's computer). Whereas professional liability protects you from claims made due to "things you do" as a practitioner, general liability protects you from claims made due to "where you work." Since personal injury can be the basis for this type of claim, and personal injury claims can be extremely expensive, be sure your general liability insurance is in full effect when you start your practice.

   Some issues to be aware of include:
   - If you rent commercial space, the area you individually occupy will be covered by your general liability policy. Common areas, such as hallways and parking lots, will be the landlord's responsibility. You may want to verify the physical areas each policy covers with your office's rental or leasing manager.

- If you plan to work from your home, check with your homeowner agent on your general liability options and property insurance. Some residential policies make allowances for business use of property, and some don't. Some homeowners' policies have an optional "rider" that can extend coverage for business use. In unusual instances, homeowners' policies become void when there is commercial use of the property. Be diligent in checking into your specific situation.

3. *Property insurance*
   This coverage pays for the loss of property as a result of specified hazards such as fire, windstorm, or theft. If you work out of your home, check your homeowners' insurance coverage. If you rent, lease, or own a separate business space, find out what kind of property insurance you will need to cover such things as loss of equipment and supplies in the event of property damage.

4. *Business interruption insurance*
   This type of coverage pays you for income lost when specified hazards prevent your practice from operating.

5. *Disability insurance*
   This type of insurance provides benefits to offset some of the income you lose if you become disabled. For most massage therapists, no work means no income. Massage therapists engage in physically demanding work - work that is often interrupted due to physical illness or injury. Disability income insurance is the type of policy that provides the disabled worker with some income when he or she can't work. Variables that affect the price include:
   - Term: How long will the policy pay benefits once benefits have begun?
   - Waiting period: How long does the beneficiary need to wait from the point of disablement until the policy starts paying benefits? The waiting period can range from 30 days to six months.
   - Benefit amount: How much of the beneficiary's income will be covered? This can range from 25 to 70 percent. Benefits are not taxable, so a 65 percent benefit is very close to actual take-home pay.
   - Type of occupation: The more likely a person's income will be disrupted due to injury, the more expensive the premium will be.
   - Age of the insured: The older the insured, the higher the premium.

6. *Workers' Compensation*
   If you employ others, you need to be aware that the government requires all businesses with at least one employee to have workers' compensation coverage. It provides comprehensive coverage to any employee who is injured on the job. Workers' compensation provides:
   - Payment of medical bills related to an on-the-job injury
   - Payment of rehabilitation services resulting from the injury
   - Payment of lost income while the employee convalesces

   You have the option to purchase workers' compensation coverage that covers yourself, but you do not need to do so. You do need to purchase coverage as soon as you employ someone.

Many people mistakenly believe that workers' compensation is a government-backed form of insurance. In fact, workers' compensation policies are issued by private insurance carriers in compliance with government regulations. Rates are based on occupational ratings. The more dangerous a job, the higher the premium. The classification of your employee and their annual earnings will determine the annual premiums.

7. *Health (medical) insurance*
   Health, or medical, insurance covers the cost of personal injury or illness. Personal medical insurance is in effect regardless of your activity that leads to the injury or illness, whereas workers' compensation covers only issues directly related to work.

   Medical insurance plans vary tremendously in cost, from low-deductible, all-inclusive (very expensive), to high-deductible, "catastrophe" plans (more affordable). As opposed to liability policies in which the insurance covers injury to others, medical insurance covers injury to the policyholder. Since injuries can be very expensive to address, purchasing medical insurance should be a very important component of your business planning.

   As a small business owner, here are some issues to be aware of:
   • You may be able to purchase personal medical insurance under a group plan. This usually means a better price but fewer options.
   • If you have workers' compensation coverage for yourself, you are only partially protected. If you break a leg skiing, you are not covered by workers' compensation.
   • Check with your accountant to see if you can claim the cost of medical insurance as a pre-tax expense in your business.
   • Medical insurance addresses your medical bills but not your lost income due to an inability to work. Only workers' compensation and disability insurance cover lost income.

   Source: Barry Antoniow. *Kiné-Concept Institute Business Success Workbook*. Fredericton, New Brunswick, Canada: Kiné-Concept Institute Maritimes.

Ask your professional association about professional and general liability coverage, plus a variety of other optional business, health, disability, term life insurance, medical and accident insurance, and business equipment and overhead insurance. You should seriously consider purchasing the optional types of insurance to protect yourself. After all, if you cannot work, you cannot practice.

Do You Need More Insurance?
Because starting a practice increases your need for insurance, review any existing policies you have with your insurance agent to learn what the policies will cover. If you need more, consult your professional association's insurance administrator for insurance options.

Remember that a homeowner's policy is designed to cover a home and its furnishings, not a business. Your homeowner's policy might cover the theft of a personal computer, because many households include one. However, you could not expect a homeowner's policy to cover the lost income that results from having to spend a week setting up a new computer system.

Massage therapists need professional liability insurance for protection against malpractice claims. In addition, contracts to work at some facilities require that you obtain extension coverage to protect the facilities from claims associated with your work there. If you need such coverage, some professional associations, such as AMTA, offer it free. You would contact the insurance administrator to set it up.

Selling Your Practice

Whatever direction your career in massage therapy takes, you may at some point decide to shift the focus of your professional life. If this happens, you may need to decide what to do with the assets of your practice. Your choices depend in part on the form of ownership you have:

- If you formed a corporation, you can sell the corporation's stock; then the new stock holder(s) own(s) your practice.
- If you formed a partnership, you and your partners can agree to dissolve the partnership (or you can leave the partnership, in which case it dissolves). Your partnership agreement will state what share of the assets each partner owns, and you are free to dispose of your assets as you see fit. Or you can find someone else to take your place in the partnership. If the other partners agree, the partnership continues without you. Finally, you and the partners can agree to sell the partnership to someone else.
- If you are a sole proprietor, you own all of the business's assets and are responsible for all of its liabilities. You can sell the assets yourself, and use them to pay off your liabilities. Another option is to sell the practice to someone else who will then operate or liquidate.

Expect that any potential buyer will want a close look at your business records so you should have them ready before you offer your business for sale. It is wise to have prospective buyers sign a confidentiality agreement so that if they decide not to go through with the purchase, any proprietary information about your business will be protected. When selling a practice, as with starting one, getting the advice of an expert (e.g. accounting, legal) will enable you to act with full understanding of tax and other implications and help you arrive at a fair deal.

Business brokers and appraisers can help you determine the value of your business. An accountant with experience in such transactions can also help you arrive at a fair selling price.

Professional Assistance

When it comes to getting professional assistance from business experts, this is a great time to start a massage therapy practice. Not only is the demand for massage growing, but so has society's appreciation of the importance of small businesses. As a result, experts in a variety of fields stand ready to help you with the technicalities of setting up and operating your practice.

Most people who start a massage therapy practice do so because they want to help others feel better through massage. However, working for yourself, either alone or in a practice with others, imposes additional responsibilities. Indeed, when you are self-employed you have to wear more than one hat. Sometimes you will wear your massage therapist's hat; at other times you will don your administrator's hat and deal with issues such as legal requirements, money, taxes, insurance, and office space.

You must become knowledgeable about many regulations and procedures in order to set up your massage therapy practice. The information is available if you spend hours in the library, on the Internet, or on the phone. However, unless you have a law degree and an accounting degree, it may be more efficient—and more wise—to call in experts in fields such as law, accounting, marketing, and graphic design.

As you plan how to set up your practice, and even after you get started, be aware of the knowledge and expertise you have, the areas you can learn quickly, and those aspects that might better be given to someone with professional training in the relevant area. To get a sense of how often you will need to seek out support services in the areas discussed previously in this chapter, complete the "Support Services" worksheet (figure 2.22, page 97) that helps you identify where you want to draw upon professional assistance, and where you want to handle the business on your own.

Where to Find Professional Assistance

You can get the most help and advice from someone who understands your situation if you work with professionals who specialize in small businesses and in the healthcare field. Try to find professionals who already have experience with other massage therapy practices. To identify such people, talk to your mentors and to other massage therapists. Ask questions such as these:

- Who is your accountant (or attorney, marketing professional, etc.)?
- How long have you used this person's services?
- In what ways has this person been helpful to you?
- Did you have any difficulty in working with this person?
- How has using this person benefited you, as opposed to doing the same work yourself?
- Do you think this person would be helpful to me? How? (Or why not?)

Figure 2.22

For each item, check whether you can and want to do it, want to learn it, or want to hire professional assistance.

	I Can and Want to Do	I Can (Want to) Learn Quickly	I Want Someone Else to Do
1. Finding out what licenses I need and what papers I must file to get started	❏	❏	❏
2. Learning the zoning laws	❏	❏	❏
3. Making sure I have a good lease for my practice space	❏	❏	❏
4. Setting up a method for keeping track of money coming in and going out	❏	❏	❏
5. Keeping my financial records up to date	❏	❏	❏
6. Preparing my tax returns and making sure I have taken all the deductions for which I am eligible	❏	❏	❏
7. Designing my logo, brochures, stationery, and business cards so that they are appealing and build a consistent image	❏	❏	❏
8. Thinking up creative ways to tell people about the benefits of my practice	❏	❏	❏
9. Writing a newsletter	❏	❏	❏

If you want someone else to do items 1–3, consider using an attorney. If you want someone else to do items 4–6, consider using an accountant. If you want someone else to do item 7, consider using a graphic designer. If you want someone else to do items 8–9, consider using a marketing communications specialist.

© 2002 American Massage Therapy Association, Evanston, IL. *The Business of Massage.* All Rights Reserved. 20026

When you have gathered two to three recommendations that sound promising, set up appointments to meet with these professionals. When you call, ask questions such as the following:

- Have you worked for other massage therapists?
- Have you worked for other organizations of my practice's size?
- Will there be a charge to meet? If so, how much?

In your meeting, ask about the professional's experience in relevant areas, such as home offices or lease negotiations. As you listen, consider whether you have good rapport with this person. If a problem occurred, would you feel comfortable calling on this person for help? After you find someone who seems well qualified and able to communicate with you, you can move on to establishing a professional relationship with him or her.

Sometimes there is a fee, because the time of a skilled professional is valuable. Some professional associations make available free legal advice to members.

Communications Strategies for Setting Up Professional Relationships

Consider whether you will want professional advice on an ongoing basis. Most massage therapists have sole proprietorships (that is, they have no partners or shareholders), so their businesses are fairly simple, and they don't need constant or frequent advice. More than likely, they simply want help getting started, preparing tax returns, finding a new location, or developing marketing materials. Thus, probably you will want to be billed only for specific tasks you request the person to do. In that case, you need to agree on what the scope of the services will be and what the professional will charge you. Be sure to agree to the services in writing before the professional begins any work for you.

Sometimes the fee for a professional service may seem high. Suppose your accountant says preparing your year-end taxes will cost $250, and you think, "But that's only for routine paperwork! I even did all the bookkeeping myself." Instead of jumping to the conclusion that the accountant's fee is too expensive, compare the fee to doing the work yourself. How long would it take you to prepare the same tax return? If you have a variety of expenses related to an office, equipment, and employees, you will need days to be sure you have prepared your returns correctly. Could you earn as much as the accountant's fee by providing massage during that same time period? And which task would you rather be doing?

Before you contact any professional to discuss your needs, you will want to be clear about what you want that individual to do for you. If you decide to interview more than one person for the same assignment, presenting a clear list of what you need will help you compare different individuals' proposals on an apples-to-apples basis.

Professional negotiators recommend getting a few written quotes for the service you request, and then comparing the quotes. This gives you some negotiating power if you want to bargain. Be sure that the person charging less is offering you services of acceptable quality and scope. Before you decide to interview and request quotes from several professionals, however, reflect on how you like to be treated by your clients and whether you find price comparisons the best way to choose a professional. You might decide to favor one professional, based on the recommendation of friends and associates, and see first whether you can negotiate an acceptable fee with that person.

Compared to the real cost of doing everything yourself, a professional's fees may look like a bargain. However, if the professional you want to work with charges fees that seem high, negotiate with him or her for something you can accept. Explain that the fee quoted is a lot of money for your practice to afford but that the professional was recommended highly, that you had hoped the fees would be less, and that you want to work out a reduced fee with him or her. The professional may be willing to be flexible about the fee, especially if you mention that as your practice grows, you will renegotiate your arrangements.

If you do not have the money to pay a professional's fee, an alternative is to explore whether the person is willing to consider a barter arrangement. With barter, no money exchanges hands. Rather, you exchange services or goods that you agree are of equal value. For example, you might agree that income tax preparation is worth two one-hour massage sessions. If you enter into barter arrangements, the value of the services you receive is considered taxable income, so the IRS requires you to declare it on your income tax return. You might be able to write off expenses you incur to fulfill your end of the barter arrangement. Always be sure to consult with your accountant about any tax-related questions. [Sohnen-Moe, Cherie. "Work Smarter with Barter." *Massage Therapy Journal*, Summer 1996, pages 149-150, 152.]

Valued Advisors

Some people are reluctant to hire an accountant or attorney because they believe they can handle the paperwork of tax returns, financial statements, and contracts themselves. That may be true, but accountants and attorneys with small-business experience do not do only paperwork; they can be valuable advisers, as well.

If you establish relationships with professionals you trust, you can consult them whenever you make a significant move, such as setting up a new location, buying a big piece of equipment, or considering an ongoing business relationship with a spa. The professionals may be aware of financial or legal implications that had not occurred to you, or they may suggest ways to protect yourself or to get the most out of your efforts.

Policy Preview

This section briefly describes the policies a practitioner needs to set up prior to opening the doors of a practice. More detailed information about deciding which policies you will establish for your business is included under "Policy Setting" (chapter 5, page 216).

Whether as an employee, a sole proprietor, or in a practice that requires managing personnel, it is best to have policies to follow. A policy is a statement of what is and is not acceptable. When you encounter a situation governed by a policy, it gives you a basis for handling the situation. For example, if your practice has a policy not to accept tips, whenever a client offers a tip you can simply reply, "No, thank you, our policy is not to accept tips."

When you establish your business, you will want to have policies in place from the beginning. You may find that you will change your policies over time, often based on client feedback, employee feedback, and your own changes in opinion about what works and what feels right. Chapter 5 discusses these policy areas in more detail.

If you have your own office, you will have wide latitude in setting policies. If you work at client sites, you will be influenced by your clients' policies, but as an independent contractor, you still will have some latitude in governing what is acceptable. Establish your policies before you look for work and discuss them when you interview. Be sure that your policies are compatible with those of the organizations at which you consider working.

"Policies for Your Business" (figure 2.23, page 101) suggests where you might want to establish formal policies. They are only a preview, as chapter 5 covers ethics, confidentiality, boundaries, communications, and other issues that influence the type of policies you might want to develop, which will help promote an appropriate therapeutic relationship between you and your clients.

When you have finished developing your policies, prepare printed versions in a manual for you and each of your employees, if any. Post important policies such as your professional association's code of ethics where you can easily refer to it. During your employee meetings, review and discuss policies periodically. Make sure everyone gets a copy, reads it, and understands it. You may even request that your employees sign a statement acknowledging they have done so.

Figure 2.23 Policies for Your Business

Business Policies
- adherence to a code of ethics
- adherence to standards of practice
- days/hours open to clients
- confidentiality between practitioners and clients
- confidentiality between practitioners and other professionals
- confidentiality between employer and employee
- fee structure
- discount policy
- complimentary massage
- acceptance of credit cards
- tipping
- safety and security

Client Policies
- customer service philosophy
- cancellation policy
- client intake forms required
- SOAP notes required
- professional boundaries between client and practitioner
- acceptance of new clients
- referrals outside of practice
- acceptance of insured clients

Employee Policies
- work hours and days
- benefits
- dress and hygiene requirements
- competition from employees
- reasons for dismissal
- pay increases and bonuses

Figure 2.24

CAREER AND PRACTICE PLANNING WORKSHEET

Page 1 of 5

Your Basic Goals and Objectives

1. What do you hope to accomplish? (What type of job are you seeking or type of practice do you want to set up?) _____

_____

2. What are your desired work hours (including massage hours per week)?_____

3. What are your objectives for income?_____

_____

4. In what time frame do you want to achieve this? _____

Background

1. How large is the demand for massage in your market? _____

2. What massage services are being provided already in your area? _____

_____

3. What is the current number of consumers already receiving massage?_____

4. How much unmet demand is there in your community?_____

5. What additional needs do you see for massage services? _____

_____

6. Of those services, what services should you plan to provide?_____

_____

7. How will your services meet the needs of the community that are not being met already?_____

_____

8. What experience, skills, and credentials do you have that will enable you to meet that need? _____

_____

_____

9. Will you be working with others? _____ If so, how will their experience and skills contribute to meeting the need you have defined? _____

_____

10. What laws and licensing requirements exist in your locale? _____

_____

11. How do you plan to comply with them?_____

_____

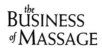

© 2002 American Massage Therapy Association, Evanston, IL. *The Business of Massage.* All Rights Reserved. #20026

12. What challenges do you expect to face in achieving your objectives, and how do you plan to overcome those challenges? _____

_____

_____

Marketing

Your Clients (Target Market)

1. What category(ies) of potential clients do you plan to serve? Define them as specifically as you can. _____

_____

2. How many clients in your area do you estimate are in each category?_____

_____

3. Is the total number of clients in these categories large enough to meet your objectives as previously stated?__

_____

4. If not, what other client category will you target, or in what other communities will you work? _____

_____

5. Might other client categories seek your services?_____ If so, who and how many?_____

_____

Your Services and Products

1. What specific massage modalities do you plan to offer? _____

_____

2. What, if any, other services (such as nutrition counseling, aromatherapy, yoga, teaching, workshops) do you plan to offer?_____ Are you already trained in or qualified to offer these? _____

_____

3. What, if any, tangible products (such as lotions, vitamins, CDs, T-shirts) do you plan to sell? _____

_____

4. How do the additional products and services fit with your main practice of massage therapy?_____

_____

_____

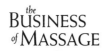

© 2002 American Massage Therapy Association, Evanston, IL. *The Business of Massage.* All Rights Reserved. #20026

Pricing

1. What price do you plan to charge for each type of service or product? For each, indicate the price charged by other local sources of the service or product:

Service/Product   My Price   Local Price

_____ _____ _____

_____ _____ _____

_____ _____ _____

_____ _____ _____

2. If your prices are different from other providers' prices, explain how you will rationalize the difference to your clients. _____

_____

_____

3. Do you plan to discount?_____ If so, how much?_____

_____

Communications

1. What will you name your business, and how will you create and communicate your business image? _____

_____

2. How do you intend to tell your targeted potential clients (or prospective employers) about your services?____

_____

3. Do you intend to have special offers? _____ If so, describe them. _____

_____

_____

Operations: Where and How You Will Practice

1. Do you plan to practice in a room in your home, at a separate office you rent or own, or at clients' (or employers') facilities?_____

_____

2. What equipment and supplies (assets) will you need to practice in that location, offering the services and products previously described? (Consider office needs, such as a desk, computer, and phone line, as well as what you need for massage therapy itself.) _____

_____

3. What other furnishings will you need to provide in order to create the desired environment for your practice?_____

_____

the BUSINESS of MASSAGE

© 2002 American Massage Therapy Association, Evanston, IL. *The Business of Massage.* All Rights Reserved. #20026

4. Who, if anyone, will work with you? _____

5. Will you be responsible for hiring or contracting with these people? _____ If so, how will you locate them? _____

_____

6. Will you be responsible for training and evaluating the people who work with you? _____
If so, how will you go about this? _____

_____

Your Financial Objectives and Plans

1. What will be your total costs of getting started? Consider the following categories:

Job-Hunting Expenses

- Printing résumés: _____
- Travel to and from interviews: _____
- Correspondence with interviewers and other networking contacts: _____
- Other: _____
- Total: _____

Practice Start-Up Expenses

- Printing business cards, stationery, brochures: _____
- Dues for professional and other organizations: _____
- Correspondence with professionals and other networking contacts: _____
- Cost of setting up office and/or practice space in home or other location (includes bringing into compliance with regulations and upgrading plumbing/electricity/ventilation): _____
- Rent (and initial deposit) for office/practice space: _____
- Purchase of equipment and supplies: _____
- Fees for professional services such as attorney or accountant: _____
- Government fees such as license, business license tax, or incorporation fees: _____
- Liability insurance: _____
- Other: _____
- Total: _____

the
BUSINESS
of MASSAGE

© 2002 American Massage Therapy Association, Evanston, IL. *The Business of Massage.* All Rights Reserved. #20026

2. Where will you obtain the funds for these job-hunting or start-up expenses? Consider your own assets, sharing ownership (equity), or borrowing (liabilities). _____

    _____

3. How much do you expect to spend each month (ongoing expenses) on each of the following:

Marketing communication: $ _____	Professional services (attorney,		
Rent/lease/mortgage: $ _____	accountant, etc.):	$ _____	
Supplies: $ _____	Taxes (property, business, income): $ _____		
Merchandise to sell: $ _____	Insurance:	$ _____	
Loan payments: $ _____	Other expenses (equipment,		
Phone and utilities: $ _____	continuing education, school		
Employees: $ _____	loans, laundry):	$ _____	
_____	Total:	$ _____	

4. What do you expect to earn each month (revenues)? From massage sessions: _____
    From product sales: _____
    From room rental to other practitioners: _____
    How soon do you think you can reach that level of earnings? _____

5. Does your expected level of revenues exceed your estimated monthly (ongoing) expenses? _____
    If not, where will you obtain funds to operate your practice? _____

    _____

6. How many massages a month must you provide in order to cover your expenses? _____

7. At your expected level of earnings and expenses, how long will it take before you have paid your start-up (or job-hunting) expenses and begun earning enough to meet your income needs? (Consider your local cost of living and the needs of yourself and family members, if any.) _____

8. How will you support yourself until you are meeting your income needs? _____

    _____

    _____

Evaluation of Your Plan

1. Do the details of your plan support the goals you defined in the first section? _____
    Explain how they do or do not support your goals. _____

    _____

2. If your plan does not fully support your goals, what changes do you need to make to your goals or your plan so that you can meet your objectives? _____

    _____

the
BUSINESS
of MASSAGE

© 2002 American Massage Therapy Association, Evanston, IL. *The Business of Massage.* All Rights Reserved. #20026

Chapter Summary

Launching your practice means putting your dreams and ideas into action. Your career as a massage therapist empowers you to make many decisions about where you will work and how your workplace will look and feel. Whether you decide to provide massage as an employee or provide it through your own business, your practice will carry its own identity in terms of your technical and client-care skills.

Creating a business plan is important because it allows you to develop short-term and long-term goals that will direct your career, whether as an employee or self-employed. After you decide on your goals, you will develop objectives that essentially give you an action plan for achieving your goals. The major sections of a business plan include: 1) your market; 2) your marketing plan; 3) your operating plan; 4) your financial plan.

In creating your business plan, you will need to learn what is required of your business in terms of local licenses and permits, zoning requirements, and insurance. If your plan includes hiring employees, you will need to understand employment laws and hiring practices. You will also want to become familiar with professional assistance that is available to you so you can decide whether you want to learn to do specialty tasks, such as bookkeeping, yourself, or to hire someone else to do it for you.

If you seek employment as a massage therapist, you would start by creating goals and objectives, just as you would do if you were starting a business. You would learn about prospective employers in your area, create your résumé and cover letters, and practice appropriate interview strategies before going on your first interview. The result of thorough planning is getting a job that helps you build a satisfying career, even if your first job is a stepping stone to a more suitable job later.

Enjoy making all the decisions required in the initial stages of launching your career, because they enable you to practice your profession in the way you have envisioned.

Review Questions

1. What are appropriate steps for launching your massage career?

2. What strategy and tools can you use to improve the effectiveness of job hunting?

3. What are the basic components of a business plan?

4. For what purposes would you use a business plan?

5. What are a few effective communications strategies that can help you build your practice?

6. What common legal issues do you need to be aware of when opening your practice?

3

MANAGING YOUR PRACTICE

CHAPTER PREVIEW:

- Financial Management

- Client Records Management

- Administrative Management

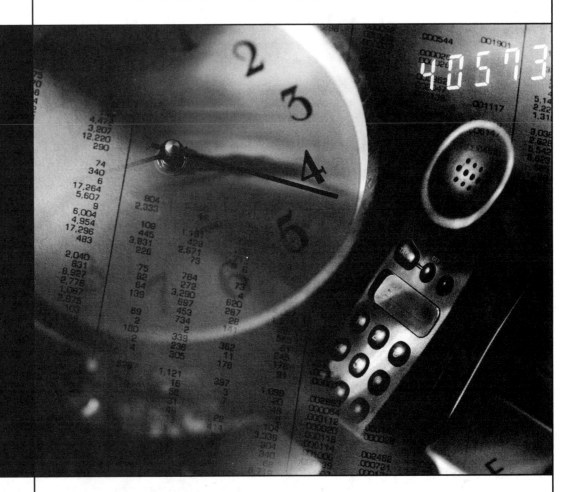

PUT GOOD MANAGEMENT SYSTEMS IN PLACE IN YOUR PRACTICE TO PROVIDE SKILLED AND NURTURING TOUCH TO CLIENTS.

Chapter Objectives

1. Identify basic business practices relevant to the management of a massage therapy practice.

2. Identify strategies for effective communication with other professionals regarding client care and referrals.

3. Identify strategies for effective management of the work environment.

4. Identify legal considerations that affect you if you have employees.

Bringing your vision of a successful massage therapy practice to life and making it profitable depends on your ability to manage it. Managing includes all the activities that ensure you are doing what you must in order to reach your goals in a way that is organized and focused. This chapter helps you by providing guidance in understanding financial records, taxes, insurance, client records, and administrative duties.

Financial Management

Good financial management is a learned skill that allows you to continue doing what you went into business for in the first place—to improve people's lives by giving them massage. Once you grasp the importance of a few key financial reports, you will appreciate how helpful they are in letting you view your practice's financial health. They will serve as your early warning system, to alert you to trends and patterns that might need to be corrected in order to become or remain profitable.

The creation of these financial reports requires regular and systematic recordkeeping. Recordkeeping can become a gratifying part of your practice when you understand the relationship of recordkeeping and its impact on increasing your profits, keeping you from getting into tax trouble, saving you time at the end of every month, and enhancing your value to clients. Invest a solid chunk of time before you open the doors of your practice to create a system of paperwork that allows you to devote minimum time to maintaining the system. The key to good recordkeeping is consistency in keeping your records updated. Those records are much easier to maintain when you've taken the time to establish a system that makes sense to you.

Creating a Budget

When you created your "Career and Practice Planning Worksheet" in chapter 2, you developed the basics for budgeting. A budget is simply a listing of the money you plan to spend, organized by expense category, and the money you anticipate receiving.

To create an expense budget, you can use a format such as "Budget Worksheet: Expenses" (figure 3.1, page 112). Complete the first worksheet, which details expenses, by following these steps:

1. List all the expenses you think you might incur in operating your practice. To prepare a complete list, review *Your Financial Objectives and Plans* in the "Career and Practice Planning Worksheet" at the end of chapter 2.
2. Organize the expenses in your list into categories, such as operations (actually providing massages or other services or selling products), marketing, administration (setting up and running your office), taxes and license fees, rent, utilities, and wages paid to employees and/or fees paid to contractors.
3. For each item in a category, estimate for each month what you will spend on that item.

4. Add the monthly amounts for each item to determine annual amounts.
5. Add the annual amounts for each item in each category to get totals for each category of expense.

It will be helpful if you maintain separate expense entries for items that directly affect your cost of providing massage, such as oils, sheets and laundry service. Expenses related to production of income are considered "cost of goods," and they should be distinguishable from expenses associated with general business activity, such as office supplies, bank charges, and telephone services. Maintaining individual budget lines for specific expenses will also allow you to compare prices to previous periods or to industry averages, so you know when to search for more competitive pricing.

You can follow a similar process to estimate all your sources of income by type of account (i.e., relaxation massage, on-site massage, third-party reimbursement). To do this, complete the worksheet "Budget Worksheet: Revenues" (figure 3.2, page 113), following the same steps as for the expense worksheet. This time, substitute the revenue categories for the expense categories. For example, you might plan to do a lot of chair (on-site) massages in stores during the December holiday shopping season, then cut back on the chair massages in January and focus on providing massages to people who received gift certificates. Estimate the total for each month and for each category of account. Then add your estimates to get totals for the year and for each category.

Many people prefer to create a budget on a computer. Once you have learned the software, it can make your work easier in many ways, including computing all your totals automatically. A variety of software programs are available to help small businesses such as yours set up budgets and compare them to actual expenses. See "Software for Financial Management" on page 114 for a list of helpful software programs.

Making Your Budget Work for You

A budget is beneficial only if you use it. There are several ways to do so:

- Create an expense and revenue budget when you are starting your practice. Review it to make sure you have enough funds to get started. If you see months when you may be short of cash, plan how you will handle that potential challenge.
- Review your budget at least once a month. Add your actual expenses for that month, as well as your total for the year so far. Are your expenses within your budget guidelines? Or, is there a need to change your spending or your budget?
- Follow a similar monthly process to evaluate whether your earnings have lived up to your expectations. If they have fallen short, how can you improve your situation? (See the "Recovery Strategies" section in chapter 7 for marketing strategies and techniques to help you.) If earnings have exceeded your expectations, has your massage practice experience been positive for you, and are you experiencing the balance you seek? Do you want to expand your practice or limit your clients?
- Create a new budget at the end of each year to plan for the following year. Then review it before you begin your new year. Will your budget enable you to meet your goals? If not, what can you change?
- Review your budget regularly. Remember that it is a guideline you have created to help you reach your goals. It is okay to change your budget if it is not getting you where you want to go.

Figure 3.1

Expense Category	Jan.	Feb.	Mar.	Apr.	May	June	July	Aug.	Sept.	Oct.	Nov.	Dec.	Total Year
Oils													
Linens													
Laundry services													
Other massage supplies													
Wages paid to employees													
Commissions and fees paid													
Employee benefit programs													
Subscriptions													
Office supplies													
Advertising													
Utilities													
Rent, lease, or mortgage													
Depreciation													
Taxes and licenses													
Travel, meals, entertainment													
Professional liability insurance													
Dues for professional organizations													
Continuing education													
Legal and professional services													
Interest payments													
Repairs and maintenance													
Car expenses													
Bad debts													
Other expenses													
Total Expenses													

the BUSINESS *of* MASSAGE

© 2002 American Massage Therapy Association, Evanston, IL. *The Business of Massage.* All Rights Reserved. #20026

Figure 3.2

Revenue Category	Jan.	Feb.	Mar.	Apr.	May	June	July	Aug.	Sept.	Oct.	Nov.	Dec.	Total Year
Relaxation massages													
Medical massages													
Sports/fitness massages													
On-site massages													
Third-party reimbursement massages													
Other massages:													
Other services:													
Rent from shared space													
Fees from employees/contractors													
Product sales													
Other revenues:													
Total Revenues													

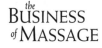

© 2002 American Massage Therapy Association, Evanston, IL. *The Business of Massage.* All Rights Reserved. #20026

Am I an Expense?

Most people who set up a massage practice intend to earn enough to live on (or contribute to their household income). That means you should include income for yourself in your budget.

If you have partners, you must allocate compensation among them. The way you will divide the partnership's income is something that you and your partners should agree on at the outset, when you prepare your partnership agreement.

Resources

Sources of Information About Software for Financial Management

- your local office supply or computer store
- product reviews in computer magazines
- product reviews in massage therapy publications
- Web board conference rooms
- your mentor and other massage therapists

Software for Financial Management

- Quicken®: www.quicken.com (for a small practice)
- QuickBooks®: www.quickbooks.com
- MYOB Limited®: www.myob.com
- Peachtree First Accounting®: www.peachtree.com
- Software is available at office supply stores and computer software stores. You can also order it online.

Financial Statements

Whether you decide to do your own accounting and bookkeeping or hire a professional to do it for you, you will at a minimum need to keep track of money that's coming into and going out of your business.

Your budget and billing records are a useful starting point for preparing financial statements, which are widely used formats for recording and evaluating how well a business is doing financially. There are three basic kinds of financial statements: balance sheets, income statements, and cash flow statements. They are important for several reasons. First, partnerships will want these statements so that all the partners can be clear about the practice's performance, and sole proprietors can benefit from preparing them to monitor their performance and identify weaknesses to correct. Second, if you incorporate, the law requires that the corporation prepare each of these statements at least once a year. And finally, financial statements are an essential part of a loan application.

The basic financial reports you should develop for your practice include:

Type of Report	Purpose of Report	Frequency
Ledger Sheets: the basis from which financial statements are created	Shows all income and expenses, categorized by type (supplies, wages, etc.)	Daily. Well-kept checking account records provide the same information as a ledger, but they are not categorized by type of expense.
Balance Sheet	Shows your practice's assets, liabilities, and equity. This is different from the income statement because it includes capital assets such as equipment you already own and lease deposits that will be refunded to you later.	Quarterly or annually
Income Statement	Shows your practice's revenues, its expenses, and its income or profit.	Monthly and year-to-date
Cash Flow Statement	Shows your practice's existing cash on hand, as well as its income and expenses.	The most helpful cash flow statement is one you create that projects your income and expenses for the month so you know if you will need to borrow money or delay expenses in order to stay in the black.

Ledger Sheets

The starting point for preparing any financial statement is to keep detailed records on ledger sheets, such as the one shown in "Ledger Sheet" (figure 3.3, page 116). A ledger sheet may be literally a sheet of paper in a book, or it may be a computer document with the same format. Your checking account record will provide the information for your ledger sheet, as it will show your payments and deposits in chronological order. To create the necessary financial statements for your business, you will want to categorize these expenses into types, such as office supplies, massage supplies, wages, rent, utilities, laundry, etc.

For revenues, record:
- the date work was performed (In places where an accrual basis of accounting is required, you must record your income when the work is performed, not when payment is received. If you are billing by invoice, such as for rent from shared space, record the date of invoice.)
- the date you received payment
- who paid you
- the invoice number
- the amount you received
- the form of payment (cash, check, charge). It is also helpful to record the check number or reference number of the charge in the event you have to track the payment later.
- year-to-date total

For expenses, record in the appropriate category (i.e., supplies, equipment):
- the date you paid
- who you paid
- what you purchased
- the check number
- the amount you paid
- the form of payment (cash, check, charge)
- year-to-date total

At the end of each month, add the entries to find the monthly total and the year-to-date amounts (how much you earned or spent so far that year). Do this regularly, to keep the task simple.

Figure 3.3 Ledger Sheet

Revenues
Type: Rent from Shared Space

Date Billed	Date Payment Received	Received From	Invoice #	Amount	Form of Payment	Yr. to Date
01-03-03	01-03-03	Jan Mulgrew	#204	$150	check #708	$150
02-03-03	02-03-03	Jan Mulgrew	#211	$150	cash	$300
03-03-03	03-03-03	Jan Mulgrew	#228	$150	check #795	$450

Expenses
Type: Office Supplies

Date Paid	Payment To	Item or Service Purchased	Check #	Amount	Form of Payment	Yr. to Date
01-03-03	Enterprise Office Supplies	3 reams paper	#704	$19.54	check	$19.54
01-18-03	Office Discount Warehouse	toner cartridge	#707	$52.19	credit card	$71.73
02-01-03	Office Discount Warehouse	business envelopes, diskettes	#710	$16.20	credit card	$87.93

Balance Sheet

A balance sheet is like a financial snapshot of your practice. As in "Simplified Balance Sheet" (figure 3.4, page 118), it shows three things:

1. *Your practice's assets*: everything you have, from cash to furniture, that you can use to operate the practice
2. *Your practice's liabilities*: everything your practice owes, such as loan payments and utility bills
3. *Your practice's equity*: the value that remains after you subtract the total liabilities from the total assets. The concept of equity reflects an accumulation of the owner's investments, withdrawals, and the accumulated earnings of your business.

Your balance sheet shows where your practice stands at the end of a particular time period, such as the end of the year or the end of a quarter.

To prepare a balance sheet, you begin by listing all the assets of the business:

- *Current assets:* The first assets to list are those you can spend within the next month, such as cash and the value of your accounts receivable (the bills you have sent out).
- *Other assets:* Next, list your other assets, including the value of your inventory (if you have items for sale), supplies, and equipment.
- *Fixed assets and depreciation:* Fixed assets—generally anything over $250 in a massage practice—are said to depreciate. A fixed asset has a useful life, and you may expense the item over the useful life of the asset. This means that each year you own the asset, you subtract part of its value. To do this, use a depreciation table or consult an accountant.
- *Total assets:* Complete the top portion of the balance sheet by adding the asset values to determine total assets.

Next, prepare the bottom half of the balance sheet:

- *Liabilities:* List the practice's liabilities, which will mainly be any bills you have not paid yet.
- *Total liabilities:* Add the liability items and record the total liabilities.
- *Owners' equity:* Subtract total liabilities from total assets. The result is equal to the owners' equity. Record this amount under the total liabilities.
- *Total liabilities and owners' equity:* Finally, add the total liabilities and the owners' equity.

If you did everything correctly, the sum of the total liabilities and owners' equity equals the total assets, thus the name "balance" sheet.

In practice, many rules govern the preparation of balance sheets and other financial statements, including the calculation of depreciation. It is up to you to decide whether you want to learn these rules or to hire an accountant.

Figure 3.4: Simplified Balance Sheet

Assets

Cash	$4,800
Accounts Receivable	400
Inventory	700
Supplies	1,000
Equipment	3,000
Total Assets	$9,900

Liabilities and Owners' Equity

Liabilities	
Accounts Payable	$1,800
Owners' Equity	
M. Johnson, Capital	8,100
Total Liabilities and Owners' Equity	$9,900

Income Statement

Besides knowing what your practice owns, you (and your lenders) will want to know whether it is making money. For this, you prepare an income statement, such as the sample in "Simplified Income Statement" (figure 3.5, page 119), which describes the practice's financial performance in terms of three basic measures:

1. *Your revenues:* the payments you received (from clients, interest on bank accounts, and so on)
2. *Your expenses:* the payments you made
3. *Your income or profit:* your total revenues minus your total expenses

By preparing an income statement after the close of each year, you can compare statements from year to year to see whether you are achieving your financial goals and building your income. If your income is not growing, you may want to make some changes to achieve your financial goals.

From your ledger sheets, you will have the information to put into the format of the income statement:

1. At the top, record your revenues by category (service or product).
2. Add your revenue amounts to find total revenues.
3. Below that number, list the expense categories and the amount for each.
4. Add the expenses to find the total expenses.
5. Record your gross profit: total revenues minus total expenses.
6. Subtract your income taxes. The result is your net profit.

If you prepare income statements, they will be very helpful when it comes time to pay quarterly estimated taxes and prepare your tax returns. If you are a sole proprietor, the basic information on an income statement corresponds to the information you will need to provide on Schedule C with your annual federal income tax return.

Figure 3.5 Simplified Income Statement

Report covers period _____ [date] to _____ [date]

Revenues

Revenue from massages	$34,000
Revenue from product sales	2,500
Fee from associate (who shares space)	5,000
Total revenues	$41,500

Expenses

Salary (part-time bookkeeper)	$5,000
Rent	9,450
Purchases of products for sale	1,500
Marketing communication	2,500
Utilities	1,000
Supplies, laundry	2,000
Membership fees, continuing education, and professional publications	2,250
Total expenses	$23,700

Net Profit (revenues minus expenses)	$17,800
Less income tax	$2,650
Net Profit after Tax	**$15,150**

Note: This example uses a 15 percent tax rate. Tax rates vary, and you should use the rate that applies to your particular situation.

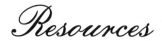

Resources

Sources of Information About How to Prepare Financial Statements

- your accountant
- Kamoroff, Bernard B. *Small Time Operator: How to Start Your Own Business, Keep Your Books, Pay Your Taxes, and Stay Out of Trouble, 25th edition.* Laytonville & Willits, CA: Bell Springs Publishing, 2000.
- Internal Revenue Service: www.irs.gov, for information about preparing statements that comply with income tax regulations
- U.S. Securities and Exchange Commission: www.sec.gov, or check the federal government listings in your phone book, for information about preparing statements that comply with rules governing how corporations report their performance

Cash Flow Statement

A common problem of many new businesses is that, although they have a lot of work to do, they keep running out of the cash they need for day-to-day expenses. To head off this problem, keep an eye on your practice's cash flow—the amount of cash received by the practice versus the amount it spends.

For a small practice, preparing a cash flow statement after-the-fact probably is less important than projecting your cash flow. A cash flow projection is like a month-by-month budget, but each item you record should involve receiving or spending cash (including checks and credit card receipts). For example, doing work for which you will bill an insurer will not generate immediate cash, but receiving the insurer's payment will in the month you receive it. Likewise, charging something on your credit card does not involve spending cash; paying the credit card bill (including interest) does. Look at each month's totals to see whether the business will generate enough cash to pay your bills that month. If it will not, you will need to plan to have some funds available when you need them (in savings, by borrowing, or by establishing a line of credit with your bank).

The formal way to do this is with a cash flow statement, such as the one in the "Simplified Cash Flow Statement" (figure 3.6, page 121). To prepare this statement, follow these steps:

1. Record the amount of cash you received during the period.
2. Record the amount of cash (including checks) you paid out for expenses (not investments, such as buying equipment).
3. Subtract total cash paid out from total cash received to find net cash from operations.
4. Record the amount of cash you received from and spent on investments, such as interest earned, equipment purchases, and stock purchases. In this example, the massage therapist purchased equipment but did not have money coming in from investments, so the only cash flow is negative—that is, money going out of the practice.
5. Record cash flows from financing. This can include investments the owner made in the business (positive cash flow) or draws by the owner (negative cash flow, because the owner takes money from the practice).
6. Add all the positive cash flows and subtract from that figure the total negative cash flows to find the net increase or decrease in cash.
7. Record the amount of cash the practice had at the beginning of the statement period. Add this to the net increase or decrease to find the cash at the end of the period.

Your cash flow statement should also include non-cash income and expense. An example of non-cash income would be accounts receivable, such as when you send an invoice to a client but have not yet received payment. An example of non-cash expense would be accounts payable, such as when you charge an item to your credit card but have not yet paid the credit card bill. These are "accrual" income and expenses, which means you have "accrued" them, or "added" them, and are important to identify in your financial statements.

Figure 3.6: Simplified Cash Flow Statement

Cash Flows from Operations for Period [month/date/year] **to** [month/date/year]

Cash receipts from revenues	$34,000
Cash payments for expenses	(5,100)
Net cash from operations	$28,900

Cash Flows from Investing

Purchase of equipment	($ 1,200)

Cash Flows from Financing

Investments by owner	$1,000
Draws by owner	(25,000)
Net Increase (or Decrease) in Cash	$3,700
Cash at the Beginning of the Period	1,800
Cash at the End of the Period	$5,500

Financial Records

Whereas budgets are projections you create before you provide services or sell goods, and financial statements are reports that help you keep your finger on the financial pulse of your business, it's the day-to-date recordkeeping that will be a testament to your financial prowess as a business owner. This section describes the types of financial records you will want to keep, and tips for maintaining them without undue stress or time commitment.

The Value of Keeping Good Financial Records

- Your clients may want or need information about their expenses. A bill from you shows what they owe, and a receipt shows what they paid. These forms also tell what products or services they received, as well as the date of the service.
- You (and your accountant) will need a record of how much you have earned and what, if anything, your clients still owe you. The amount they owe is an asset of your practice.
- The Internal Revenue Service requires receipts for deductions.
- If you apply for a loan, your probability of being approved could depend on the accuracy and reliability of your financial records.

Invoices

The most basic kind of billing record is a copy of your bill. A bill—also called an invoice—is a request for payment. Your bill, as shown in "Invoice" (figure 3.7, page 123), should include the following information:

- the name, address, and phone number of your practice (as on your letterhead)
- your registration or license number
- the invoice date and number
- the name of the client
- the date you provided services or sold goods, if different from the date of the bill

- a description of the services provided and products sold (for example, "1-hour massage" or "aromatherapy pillow")
- the cost of each item and the total amount due (indicating the amount of sales tax separately, if any applies)
- a statement of finance terms, e.g., "Payment due upon receipt of invoice."
- expression of appreciation for their business

When your client pays, you can mark the bill "paid in full" and use a copy as a receipt for the client. A receipt is a document showing that the person billing has received payment.

There are some variations. If you contract with a spa, health club, health clinic, or other organization, your contract will determine whether you will bill for the number of massages, time with clients, or some other arrangement. Your bill would detail how you fulfilled the contract (for example, "10 hours at x dollars per hour"). Also, if you are billing a third-party payer, such as an insurance company, the payer will probably have some requirements about the information you provide. (Third-party reimbursement is covered in more detail on pages 159-164.)

If you are billing individual clients, you will probably bill and collect from them just after the massage. The usual way to do this is to present the bill, collect payment, and give the client a receipt in the form of the bill with a notation that you have received payment in full. If you prefer a manual method, a sales receipt book with carbon copies works great. Give the original or top copy to your client as a receipt, and keep the bottom copy as a record of payment. Computer software offers another way to keep these records. Enter the same information directly into your computer, printing out a combination bill/receipt for the client. Sales receipt books and basic software that can handle billing are available from office supply stores.

Mailing and Collecting on Invoices

If you are working under contract with organizations, such as third-party payers or organizations that provide their clients with massages, you probably will need to mail invoices. At a minimum, keep copies in an A-to-Z follow-up file folder; use a formal accounts receivable register for a large practice. When you receive a payment, make a record of when you received it. Also record the payment in your accounts receivable ledger.

Check your revenue ledger weekly to make sure your clients are paying you within about thirty days. If not, you should call the client, ask to speak with the person who handles accounts payable, and discuss the client's payment policy. If you ask questions in a professional, courteous manner, the person you talk to should be able to clarify what you can expect. If you find, for example, that insurance claims routinely take weeks to process, you can plan for the lag time or choose to focus on building a different kind of client base. Immediately after your conversation, make notes of what you learned or agreed to, so that you can refer to them the next time you review your tickler file.

Figure 3.7   INVOICE

business stamp here

CLIENT:
Name: _____   Invoice Date: _____
Address: _____   Invoice #: _____
Phone: _____   Practitioner: _____
Social Security #: _____

Date of Service	Description of Services/Products	Price	Quantity	Tax	Total Due	Payment Amount	Payment Method	Balance Due

For clients who plan to submit insurance claim:

Insurance Carrier: _____

Policy/Group #: _____

CPT CODE: _____

Referring Physician: _____

Payment due upon receipt of invoice.
We appreciate your business.

© 2002 American Massage Therapy Association, Evanston, IL. *The Business of Massage*. All Rights Reserved. #20026

the
BUSINESS
of MASSAGE

What to Do If You Do Not Get Paid

If you work primarily for clients who pay you at the time of service, you may never encounter a nonpaying client. However, if you want to work for organizations in situations in which you submit a bill and wait for payment, there is some risk of slow payment or none at all. Most organizations want to keep current with bill payment, so a polite phone call will resolve most problems. If the client has trouble paying, however, focus on setting up a payment plan—not just on demanding payment in full.

But what if patience and a phone call do not work? Consider your options, and remember that bill collection will take time. If your bill is under $100, consider whether you would be better off financially to spend that time working for another client. (Talk to your accountant about tax deductions for bad debts and collection expenses.) If the unpaid bill is large, you can contact a collection agency, which may handle collection efforts in exchange for a percentage of the fee. You certainly want to avoid angry discussions with (former) clients, and you probably will not want to take the matter to court, because it is extremely time consuming and usually expensive.

Keep your perspective. Most clients will pay, and you need to focus on your ultimate goals.

Save Your Receipts!

As you record your revenues and expenses, file all your receipts and check stubs. Sort expense receipts by category and revenue receipts (check stubs) by client type or date, so that you can easily find them again if you need to refer to them. Canada requires that all records be kept for seven years. In the United States, rules for how long you must save your records varies by document. They are shown in "Retention Guidelines for Business Records" (figure 3.8, page 125).

In judging how much information to keep and how much to throw away, it's helpful to understand retention guidelines for business records. As a general rule, you should keep:
- for five years—general correspondence
- for seven years—all tax-related information (such as returns, receipts, and records that support tax deductions, W-2s, and 1099s)
- indefinitely—all records related to tax deductions and all documentation regarding legal matters

Activity Log

Besides recording the amount of money you are owed and paid, keep track of the hours you spend earning that money. For example, using a notebook or your computer, keep a record of the number of hours you spend giving massages to each type of client.

You can use this information to compare the financial impact of serving different client types (for example, sports massage clients versus clients seeking pain relief, or private-pay clients versus insurance clients). Divide your total earnings for serving the type of clients in a particular week or month by the number of hours you spent on that client type (including travel time). Do you earn more per hour from some types of clients than from others? Is it worth your time to continue working with all types?

Figure 3.8: Retention Guidelines for Business Records

Document	Retention
General correspondence	5 years
Bank statements	7 years
Cash receipts	7 years
Cancelled checks	7 years for most (but keep cancelled checks of major purchases indefinitely)
Year-end financial statements	Indefinitely
Employee contracts	Indefinitely
Vendor contracts	Indefinitely
Licenses and permits	Indefinitely
Insurance claims	Indefinitely
Tax returns	Indefinitely

Streamline Your Recordkeeping

To know where your money comes from and where it goes, you must do careful recordkeeping. Your checkbook register is one of your most basic records. In addition, you should keep track of your expenses by category (postage, rent, phone, etc.) and of your earnings by client and by goods sold.

Software programs are useful for recording daily, weekly, or monthly revenues and expenses. With a computer, you can tailor a spreadsheet to your needs, but it is easier to buy software designed for financial records. Compare financial software features and consider which appeals most to your knowledge, preferences, and needs. Do not base your selection solely on the price of the software, because the more helpful the software is to you in designing and maintaining good financial systems, the more benefit you will gain from it.

If you are just starting out or your practice is small, or if you simply prefer to keep manual records, you can buy a three-column ledger book from an office supply store. Either way, collect the information for your income statement by setting up a page for each category of revenue and expense.

Keeping Financial Records

If you make a habit of careful recordkeeping, you will be better organized and more able to focus on your own needs and those of your clients. Here are some ways to keep good business records:

- Pay only business-related expenses with your business checking account; pay personal bills with your personal checking account.
- Devote one credit card solely to business use. (The card can be in your name or that of the practice.)
- Keep a record of every deposit to your account, as well as every payment.
- Make all deposits of business income to your business account. Depending on your type of business, you can either transfer money to your personal account or pay yourself a salary.
- For every expense, keep a record of who you paid, the amount of payment, the type of expense, and the date.
- Keep each year's appointment book or calendar with your tax records for that year. You may need to use it for backup information about business travel and related expenses.
- Billing records can also help you figure out which kinds of clients are most profitable. You can use that information to refine your marketing plans.
- The Internal Revenue Service and state tax agencies expect you to keep records of your sources and amounts of income. If you are ever audited, these agencies will inspect billing records along with your practice's other financial records.

Good billing records are also helpful in providing information to others who need to know about the business aspects of your practice (for example, lenders or buyers of the practice).

Tips for Keeping Records

Set up files to keep your important papers organized. Look through an office supply catalog to find ways to organize different kinds of records. Records to maintain and keep in a safe place include the following:

- Receipts for every expense related to your practice (filed alphabetically according to type of expense)
- Records of your appointments (organized by date)
- Copies of the receipts you issue to clients for payments, showing any sales tax you collected (organized by date)
- Copies of your tax returns dating back at least seven years

Back It Up!

If you keep records on your computer, be sure you get in the habit of saving and backing up your work. Most software programs have a quick command you use to save your data periodically. A good habit is to use the save command every five or ten minutes as you work. Then, when you finish a work session, insert a back-up disk into your computer's disk drive and make a copy of any file you were using. When you complete a report, print out the file, including the date and file name.

Although following this procedure may seem like too much trouble, everyone who avoids the task has learned at one time or another how frustrating it is to lose a day's work to a thunderstorm or brownout.

Recordkeeping can make your practice run more smoothly, or it can be an endless source of frustration. To be sure you set up the right recordkeeping procedures for your practice, you may want to consult with an accountant. Even a short meeting can generate a lot of helpful advice. You can also set up systems that will generate the forms of information that an accountant can easily work with (and that will enable you to meet IRS guidelines when you file your tax returns).

Hire a Bookkeeper

You may also want to hire a bookkeeper. The considerations listed in "Pros and Cons of Using a Bookkeeper" (figure 3.9, page 128) will help you decide whether to do so. Unlike Certified Public Accountants, bookkeepers may not be qualified to give you advice, but they can handle the day-to-day responsibility of recording the practice's transactions. Unless your practice is very large, you will not need a full-time bookkeeper. You can find someone with a good track record by getting referrals from other massage therapists or business owners in your area. Because honesty and accuracy are so essential in this line of work, be sure to ask for references and check them carefully.

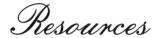

Sources to Help You Put Recordkeeping on a Computer

- courses at your local community college
- your mentor
- your accountant or attorney
- your local computer store
- Placencia, Jose, Bruce Welge, and Don Oliver, *Business Owner's Guide to Accounting & Bookkeeping.* Grants Pass, OR: The Oasis Press, 1997.
- Kamaroff, Bernard B. *Small Time Operator: How to Start Your Own Business, Keep Your Books, Pay Your Taxes, and Stay Out of Trouble,* 25th edition. Laytonville & Willits, CA: Bell Springs Publishing, 2000.
- Small Business Administration: 1-800-8-ASK-SBA; www.sba.gov

Figure 3.9: Pros and Cons of Using a Bookkeeper

Pros	*Cons*
You can delegate tasks to someone who enjoys accounting.	You are less familiar with the practical details of your practice.
Ideally, the person doing the bookkeeping is someone skilled at this type of activity, saving you time and reducing the potential for errors.	You are responsible for ensuring that the bookkeeper is honest and the figures correct. For example, you should review a week's postings every month.
You can devote your time to massage and other more productive or satisfying activities.	You must pay the bookkeeper for his or her work (in cash or through a barter arrangements). Keep in mind that barter is taxable income and you must pay taxes on the value of the service received, even if you "pay" for it with a massage.

Keeping Track of Your Money

Good business practices that keep a record of income and expenses are particularly important for credit information. To keep track of your money, you need a safe place to hold it and a system for maintaining records.

Opening a Checking Account

The simplest, safest, and most convenient place for most of your money is in a checking account at your local bank or credit union. Often, community banks are the most friendly toward a small business, such as a massage therapy practice. Make an appointment with a banker, and bring in the business plan you developed in chapter 2. It can be helpful to get to know a banker, in case you have questions or your banking needs expand as you go along.

You can negotiate terms for your banking relationships, just as you do for other professional relationships. What is the best arrangement the bank or credit union can offer you? Ask questions:

- What interest rate does this account pay on balances?
- Is there a minimum balance?
- What fees are charged if I go below the minimum balance?
- When is interest credited?
- What other fees is this account subject to?
- What are the bank's terms for setting up my account to accept payment by credit card?
- Does this account offer access to automated teller machines (ATMs)? If so, where are they? Are there fees for using them?
- Does this account offer overdraft protection? If so, how does it work?
- If I keep more money in this account, could I arrange more favorable terms?

Bank Fees

When you are comparing checking accounts, consider the fees banks typically charge. Here are some examples:

- Check printing fees
- Credit card fees
- Credit card scanner fees (if you accept payment by credit card)
- ATM fees
- Deposit fees
- Lock box drop fees
- Insufficient funds fees
- Some banks attract customers with no-fee accounts.

Two Accounts Are Better Than One

For any practice, including a sole proprietor, it is best to open a business checking account separate from your personal account. Separating your accounts will allow you to keep track of your revenues and expenses, and it will simplify your bookkeeping and financial reporting. When you earn more than enough to cover your business expenses, you can pay yourself with a draw—that is, by transferring money from your business checking account into your personal checking account.

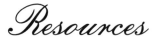

Where to Find a Bank or Credit Union
- A good place to start is the bank or credit union that handles your personal funds.
- Get references from your mentor(s), other massage therapists, business owners, and other people you know.
- Get references from your accountant or attorney.
- Look for institutions that position themselves as community banks serving local needs.

Taxes

At any gathering of massage therapist business owners, the topic of taxes is sure to generate lively discussion, because there are many war stories about practitioners who got into trouble because they didn't understand the rules for paying taxes. Understanding what is required of your business for taxes and relying on a knowledgeable accountant or tax advisor is indispensable to the financial success of your business.

If you are employed, your employer withholds taxes for you, and you do not have to file quarterly estimated taxes. Your employer already withholds federal, state, FICA (Social Security), and Medicare taxes from your pay, and gives you a W-2 form at the end of the year so you can file income tax. If you are self-employed or if you are an independent contractor, and if you earn more than $400 a year, you must pay your own federal, state, FICA, Medicare, and self-employment tax, and must file quarterly estimated taxes in April, June, September, and January, using a 1040 form. If your practice is incorporated, you must also file a corporate tax return. (The corporate return for quarterly reports of tax withholding is IRS Form 941.)

As a general rule, IRS regulations require that you pay at least 90 percent of the amount due for that quarter, or 100 percent of the amount you paid for that quarter in the previous year. If you pay less on your estimated taxes, you will owe a penalty when you file your annual return. To avoid the penalty, either pay as much as you did the preceding year or multiply your tax rate by the gross profit on your income statement.

If you have always been an employee, and if you are used to getting money back when you file your tax return every year, being self-employed will take some getting used to.

When you start your business, you will have to guess at what your total tax liability will be. Until you have an established history, err on the side of caution. A good general rule is to set aside one-third of your gross receipts for taxes, at least until you have an established record of your business's finances.

Shared Wisdom

"Don't assume you do not have to pay quarterly taxes your first year of self-employment. If you wait until the end of the tax year you may find that if you owe taxes for your self-employment earnings, you will also owe penalties. If you owed $1000, for example, IRS would expect you to pay $250 to them each quarter. If you wait and pay it all at the end of the year, you will owe penalties for paying the first quarter 10 months late and the second quarter seven months late and the third quarter four months late! It is worth the money and time to talk to an accountant as you set up your business to avoid these mistakes."

—Peggy Smith, BMSI Institute, Overland Park, Kansas

FICA

When you're an employee, your employer takes out half, and you pay the other half. When you're self-employed, you pay the entire amount. This amount constitutes a self-employment tax, and the intention is that this amount should fund your Social Security account for your later benefit.

Self-Employment Tax

In addition to the Social Security self-employment tax at the federal level, some states also apply a surcharge to self-employed individuals.

Profit & Loss

If you make a profit, you are taxed on that profit. Therefore, if you are in a position that allows you the luxury of investing profits back into your business, doing so will reduce your tax liability. For instance, if you need to buy new office furniture, it's a good idea to buy it toward the end of the tax year. Doing so enables you to invest your money for most of the year, and then to take advantage of whatever tax deductions might be allowed for business expenses in that tax year. Profit shows up on your Form 1040 as income.

Sales Tax

Some states have a sales tax on the sale of services, and many states tax the sale of goods. Some cities and counties also have sales taxes. You are responsible for determining whether the services or goods you sell are subject to sales tax. You must collect the tax at the time of service or sale and pay it according to the schedule set by the appropriate governmental body. You may also need to obtain a sales tax (or seller's) permit. In Canada, this is called the Goods and Services Tax (GST).

Income

Keep track of all income, including tips. Always issue a receipt to a client, and write "check" or "cash" on the receipt. Note the amount of tip either on the receipt or next to the client's name in the appointment book. You will need documentation that shows that your income receipts equal your bank deposits.

Do not assume that it's all right to not report tips. Some industries, such as the restaurant industry, are required by the Internal Revenue Service to automatically withhold taxes on employees' wages plus 10 percent, assuming a certain level of tips.

Understand the distinction between tax avoidance and tax evasion. Tax avoidance means that you claim something as a deduction, which might be allowed or disallowed by the IRS. If the IRS disallows the deduction, you must pay the tax plus a penalty or interest for not having paid the tax initially. Tax avoidance is not illegal. If you sell products, you also pay state sales tax that you have collected on your sales, if your state has sales tax.

Tax evasion is illegal. It means that you have not reported all of your income to the IRS, and it could result in your going to prison. Report your tips!

Deductions

In general, an expense is deductible if it meets three conditions established by the IRS:
1. You incurred the expense in connection with your practice.
2. The expense is ordinary (common or accepted as an expense of running a massage therapy practice) and necessary (appropriate or helpful for developing and maintaining your practice).

3. The deduction is based on precedent and on the reasonable belief that it is accurate.

Some deductions, such as transportation expenses and expenses for entertaining clients, are limited, however, so check with the IRS, your state tax agency, or your accountant if you are not sure about a deduction. See "Tax Deductions for a Practice" (figure 3.10, page 133) and "Special Case Tax Deductions," (figure 3.11, page 134).

Also see "Automobile Mileage Log" (figure 3.12, page 135) for an example of how you might keep track of the miles you drive for business. By securing such a log with rubber bands to your car's visor and sticking a pen under one side, you will have a recordkeeping chart handy where you can read the odometer.

Keep receipts for everything. Set up a series of file folders, label them by categories such as dues, rent, and utilities, and file the receipts in these folders as soon as you pay the expense. Putting together your tax records at the end of the year will be so much easier if you don't have to search for receipts.

It is essential to keep records of tax-related activities. Whenever you complete a tax return of any kind, keep a copy of it in your files. If you file amendments to the return, keep copies. If the IRS or state tax agency sends you any correspondence about your taxes, keep a copy in your files.

In general, it is prudent to store copies of your tax documents and supporting materials (such as receipts) for about seven years. This is especially significant for massage therapists with a home office. Tax returns with deductions for home office expenses are more likely to be audited than returns without this expense.

What Forms Do You Need?

Individual cases vary, so check with your accountant, the IRS, or the state taxing body. Listed here are the key forms required by the U.S. Internal Revenue Service for federal income taxes:

- Form 1040 for paying estimated taxes (Form 941 if you are incorporated)
- Form 1040 for calculating the tax you owe on your earnings as the operator of your sole proprietorship, a partner in your partnership, or the employee of your corporation
- Schedule C for calculating the earnings of your sole proprietorship or Schedule K1 (Form 1065) for calculating the income of your partnership. Schedule C accompanies your personal Form 1040. The managing partner of a partnership sends Schedule K1, which instructs you where to insert amounts on your Form 1040. (If your practice is incorporated, the corporation files Form 1120 to report its income.)
- Schedule SE for calculating your self-employment tax (for Social Security and Medicare), if you have a sole proprietorship or partnership
- Form W-2 for reporting the income of any employees
- Form 1099-MISC for reporting payments of $600 or more to independent contractors
- Form A for Business Use of Automobile

You may need to file other forms as well; for example, if you have property to depreciate or if you have a home office, the IRS requires additional paperwork. The "Tax Obligation Worksheet" (figure 3.13, page 136) can help you keep track of what types of taxes you need to pay and when you need to pay them.

Figure 3.10 TAX DEDUCTIONS FOR A PRACTICE

Note: The inclusion of an item on this list does not mean that it is necessarily appropriate as a business tax deduction. You need to consult with your accountant, tax advisor, or the IRS on all questions of appropriate deductions.

❏ Supplies for office and massages (i.e., bottled water, postage, lotions, music, office supplies)

❏ Cost to acquire items you offer for sale

❏ Membership dues in professional organizations

❏ Subscriptions to professional journals

❏ Subscriptions to magazines provided to clients in waiting room

❏ Fees for accountant, attorney, graphic designer, etc.

❏ Credit card fees

❏ Bank account fees

❏ Wages for employees or fees paid to contractors (deduct your own salary if your business is a corporation but not if a sole proprietorship)

❏ Telephone charges

❏ License fees

❏ Property tax, sales tax, business tax

❏ Depreciation of fixed assets (such as building and equipment)

❏ Rent/mortgage payments

❏ Utilities for office space

❏ Linen and/or cleaning service

❏ Uniforms (if a condition of employment)

❏ Gifts to clients

❏ Travel expenses and mileage related to your practice (except to and from home and your primary place of business)

❏ Meals (limited) with other professionals during which business is discussed

❏ Home office expenses (if home office is principal place of business)

❏ Insurance

❏ Attendance at professional conferences

❏ Continuing education to maintain professional credentials or expand business potential

❏ Books related to health education and massage therapy

Adapted from "Get It Together for the Accountant," by Lu Bauer. *MASSAGE THERAPY JOURNAL*®, Spring 1999, pages 79–80, 82.

the
BUSINESS
of MASSAGE

© 2002 American Massage Therapy Association, Evanston, IL. *The Business of Massage.* All Rights Reserved. #20026

Figure 3.11

SPECIAL CASE TAX DEDUCTIONS

Note: The inclusion of an item on this list does not mean that it is necessarily appropriate as a business tax deduction. Consult with your accountant, tax specialist, or the Internal Revenue Service on all questions of appropriate deductions.

Mileage

❑ IRS Form A is for Business Use of Automobile. The form specifies that you have a mileage log.

❑ Keep a mileage log that shows when/why of mileage.

❑ Get a receipt for tolls.

❑ You cannot claim mileage from home to your office as a deduction.

❑ If your business is located in your home, and you make outcalls, you cannot claim the first leg of mileage from home to the first client. You may claim mileage between second and third clients, etc., but you cannot claim from last client to home.

❑ Plan your day wisely – Make your first leg of a trip from home to a nearby business stop, such as your bank, and then make your longer business drives. End your day with a stop at, say, the post office, again closer to home.

Travel

❑ For business-related travel, including continuing education, you may deduct airfare, cab fare, hotel, registration fee, and some meals. Ask your accountant to clarify rules for meals.

Home Office

❑ Calculate percentage of square feet used solely for business.

❑ Deduct same percentage of rent/mortgage, interest, insurance, repairs and maintenance, utility bills, and property taxes.

❑ Be aware that claiming a deduction for a home office is a red flag for audits. Make sure your accountant approves all deductions. Make sure your city permits and licenses are all up-to-date, such as city occupancy permit to use home as business, establishment license, fire inspection, and property inspection.

© 2002 American Massage Therapy Association, Evanston, IL. *The Business of Massage.* All Rights Reserved. #20026

Figure 3.12

Automobile Mileage Log[1]

Date	Starting Mileage	Ending Mileage	Total Business Miles	Total Personal Miles	Total Commute[2] Miles	From	To	Reason
Page Total								

[1] Consult a tax specialist to learn when you can and cannot claim miles as a tax deduction. [2] Commute miles = distance from home to office and back home.

-------- Fold here to fit car visor. --------

Automobile Mileage Log[1]

Date	Starting Mileage	Ending Mileage	Total Business Miles	Total Personal Miles	Total Commute[2] Miles	From	To	Reason
Page Total								

[1] Consult a tax specialist to learn when you can and cannot claim miles as a tax deduction. [2] Commute miles = distance from home to office and back home.

the BUSINESS *of* MASSAGE

© 2002 American Massage Therapy Association, Evanston, IL. *The Business of Massage.* All Rights Reserved. #20026

Figure 3.13   TAX OBLIGATION WORKSHEET

Contact each area of government to inquire about the tax obligations of your practice, that is, whether you must pay a particular tax. If you must pay the tax, learn the payment date or schedule. As you collect this information, check the corresponding boxes and record your tax obligations.

Type of Tax	When Payments Are Due
Income Tax	
❑ Federal	_____
❑ Social Security (FICA) and Medicare (self-employment tax)	_____
❑ State/Province	_____
❑ County	_____
❑ City	_____
Sales Tax (Ask whether a permit is required.)	
❑ State/Province (on services? goods?)	_____
❑ County (on services? goods?)	_____
❑ City (on services? goods?)	_____
❑ GST (Goods & Services Tax) - Canada	_____
Business Taxes and License Fees	
❑ State/Province	_____
❑ County	_____
❑ City	_____
Property Taxes (on property you own and use for your practice)	
❑ State/Province	_____
❑ County	_____
❑ City	_____

Note: If you incorporate and/or hire employees, you will also have to withhold (and pay) taxes from each employee's paycheck.

the
BUSINESS
of MASSAGE

© 2002 American Massage Therapy Association, Evanston, IL. *The Business of Massage.* All Rights Reserved. #20026

Using the Services of a Professional Accountant

Unless you are particularly knowledgeable about taxes, finances, and the rules that apply to businesses, there are many advantages to hiring a professional accountant. A good accountant can help you set up efficient financial recordkeeping systems that will ultimately increase the value of your business by highlighting areas of vulnerability so that you can take corrective action. A specialist might also help prevent your business from paying higher taxes than necessary, and reduce the chance of your being audited. The time you could spend learning and doing financial and tax-related work otherwise could be spent giving massages and bringing in revenue!

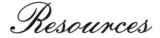

Where to Find Information About
Filing Tax Returns

- your accountant or tax advisor
- your state's tax agency
- Internal Revenue Service: 1-800-829-1040; www.irs.gov
- Revenue Canada: 1-800-267-5177; www.ccra-adrc.gc.ca
- Bernard B. Kamoroff, *Small-Time Operator: How to Start Your Own Small Business, Keep Your Books, Pay Your Taxes and Stay Out of Trouble!* Laytonville & Willits, CA: Bell Springs Publishing, 2000.

Client Records Management

You not only want to keep information about your money, but about your clients as well. Client records allow you to manage your business effectively, provide some measure of legal protection, and most importantly, provide one of the most effective mechanisms for communicating clearly with your client within the therapeutic relationship. More information about the significance of these documents to the client-practitioner relationship is contained in the "Confidentiality" section of chapter 5.

Client records will help you provide appropriate care. You will need several kinds of records, identified in "Client Records" (figure 3.14, pages 139-140). It is important to keep accurate and comprehensive records on all of your clients, including records of types of clients, money due and received, and follow-up done with clients and insurance companies.

Some client records may be consolidated onto one form rather than on separate documents. For example, the form shown in "Client Intake Form" (figure 3.15, pages 142-143) includes an informed consent statement as well as a release of medical records authorization. You may opt to exclude this section from your client intake form and offer instead separate authorization forms for these specified purposes, such as in the "Informed Consent Simplified Form" (figure 3.16, page 144) and the "Client Release of Information Form" (figure 3.17, page 145).

Keeping Client Records

Set up files to keep your important papers organized. Look through an office supply catalog to find ways to organize different kinds of records. Records to maintain and keep in a safe place include the following:

- receipts for every expense related to your practice (filed alphabetically according to type of expense)
- records of your appointments (organized by date)
- copies of the receipts you issue to clients for payments, showing any sales tax you collected (organized by date)
- client information, such as client intake form, authorization to release information, etc.

Client Intake Form

At the beginning of a client's first visit, you should devote about ten to fifteen minutes to an intake interview. During this time, gather information about your client's expectations and desired outcome from the massage therapy session. Ask the client to complete an intake form giving personal data and insurance information. The client should sign the contract for care, assignment of benefits, and release of medical records, if necessary, as well as the consent for care. Also use this form to record the client's health history. Your intake form should be designed to uncover conditions that will help you plan the course of the massage therapy session or signal your need to refer the client to his or her doctor before beginning massage therapy. For example, the health history should ask about the location and intensity of any pain, as well as numbness and swelling. See "Client Intake Form" (figure 3.15, pages 142-143).

Informed Consent Agreement

Informed consent agreements are basic to ethical standards within the massage therapy profession. They provide accurate information to clients regarding professional services offered, they help define the therapeutic and healthcare relationship, they present the credentials of the therapist and the manner in which sessions are conducted. The information enables the client to make an informed decision about whether he or she wants to receive the services. Informed consent also serves as a protective mechanism safeguarding the therapist in the event of any liability issues that may arise during or after services are provided.

Informed consent serves the needs of both the client and the therapist who have mutual responsibility for a therapeutic partnership. The client has the right to have professional services and credentials explained, as well as the responsibility to respect the business practices of the professional and to actively participate in the healing work. The therapist has the right to know information about the client in order to determine whether or not the therapeutic service will be of assistance to her or him, and the responsibility to inform the client of the benefits, limitations, contraindications, and possible outcomes of the work. [Source: Suzanne Torrenzano. "Sound Ethical Practices: Informed Consent." *Virginia In Touch*, AMTA Virginia Chapter Newsletter, June 1999.]

Figure 3.14

CLIENT RECORDS

page 1 of 2

Record	Information on Record
Informed consent agreement	❑ Information about your approach to massage, modality, and techniques ❑ Benefits, limitations, and contraindications ❑ Possible outcomes (with no promises) ❑ The nature of a session, including the process of disrobing and draping ❑ Scope of practice—what you can and cannot do given your credentials and place of business practice ❑ Your credentials and areas of expertise ❑ Session duration and fees ❑ Insurance reimbursement capabilities ❑ Availability and hours of operation ❑ Collaboration policies with other health professionals ❑ Policies for missed appointments and late arrivals ❑ Client forms to be completed
Client intake form	❑ Personal data (address, phone number, etc.) ❑ Insurance information, if necessary ❑ Health history (including previous massage therapy) ❑ Desired results from massage ❑ Informed consent (consent for care—description of the nature of massage and scope of expected benefits and risks, signed by client) ❑ Medical release authorization ❑ Assignment of benefits (payment responsibility) ❑ Contract for care (agreement to participate as part of the healthcare team)

the
BUSINESS
of MASSAGE

© 2002 American Massage Therapy Association, Evanston, IL. *The Business of Massage.* All Rights Reserved. #20026

Client release of information	❏ If medical release authorization is not included on client intake form, you may use a separate document
	❏ Name of business/clinician to whom client has requested information be sent
	❏ Address and telephone of business/clinician
	❏ Statement requesting and authorizing release of records and/or authorizing discussion of client's information with named business/clinician
	❏ Client's name, date of birth, social security number
	❏ Patient's signature and date form is signed
	❏ If authorization should span a period of time, specify "good through" date
SOAP notes	❏ **Subjective** complaints and functional goals, including information from intake form and pain questionnaire, drawing showing location of symptoms, description of any relevant injuries or surgeries (client completes)
	❏ **Objective** information from visual observation (including postural analysis), palpation, range-of-motion testing; nature of massage therapy provided
	❏ **Assessment**, including records of assessment by physician and massage therapist's documentation of subjective and objective changes that are an immediate result of the care provided
	❏ **Plan** for massage frequency, focus, and modality; recommended homework, exercises
Client telephone log	❏ Notes about how client is feeling on day after session
	❏ Follow-up log
Client visits and billing record	❏ Client name
	❏ Invoice number and date
	❏ Nature of visit
	❏ Amount billed
	❏ Date and amount of payment received

the
BUSINESS
of MASSAGE

© 2002 American Massage Therapy Association, Evanston, IL. *The Business of Massage*. All Rights Reserved. #20026

You may want to call this agreement an Informed Consent Agreement, or it could also be called a Professional Policies and Procedures agreement. It could be an attachment to the client intake form, or a separate form. Make it a practice to ask the client to arrive about 10 minutes before the scheduled appointment to complete standard health forms. After reviewing this form with the client, and making sure you have addressed any questions the client asks, write a couple of sentences at the bottom of the form specifying that the client understands the nature of the work and agrees to receive services. Include a place for the client's signature and date. See "Informed Consent Simplified Form" (figure 3.16, page 144).

For further discussion of the ethical dimensions of informed consent and their impact on your therapeutic relationship with the client, see the "Informed Consent" section in chapter 5.

Release of Information Agreement

Your client should sign a release of information agreement when he or she requests that you send information to another person or business, such as a physician or an insurance company. If medical release authorization is not included on client intake form, you may use a separate document. It should contain the following information:

- name of business/clinician to whom client has requested information be sent
- address and telephone of business/clinician
- statement requesting and authorizing release of records and/or authorizing discussion of client's information with named business/clinician.
- client's name, date of birth, Social Security number
- patient's signature and date form is signed
- If authorization should span a period of time, specify "good through" date.

See the "Health Insurance Portability and Accountability Act—HIPAA" section (page 161) for more details about confidentiality and release of client information. See "Client Release of Information Form" (figure 3.17, page 145).

Figure 3.15

Name _____ Date _____ Date of Birth _____
Phone-Work _____ Home _____ E-mail _____
Address _____ City _____ State _____ Zip _____
Occupation _____ Employer _____
Work Responsibilities _____
Primary Care Provider _____ Phone _____ Fax _____
Address _____ City _____ State _____ Zip _____
Emergency Contact _____ Relationship _____
Phone-Work _____ Home _____ Cell/Pager _____

Current Health

Have you ever received massage therapy before? __ Yes __ No   Frequency: _____
Reason for today's visit: _____
Desired results of today's session: _____
Today's primary concern or goal: _____ Other: _____
Classify concern: __ Minor __ Problematic __ Major
Classify type: __ Recurring __ Getting worse __ Getting better
Have you had this concern/goal before? __ Yes __ No   Explain: _____
Have you received treatment for this before? __ Yes __ No   Explain: _____
List activities affected: _____
Current medications: _____
(include over-the-counter pain relievers and herbal remedies)
Stress reduction/exercise activities: _____ Frequency: _____

Check any of the following that apply to your current health:
__ pregnancy   __ heart conditions   __ circulatory conditions   __ blood clots   __ diabetes
__ infections   __ cancer   __ difficulty breathing   __ arthritis
Comments: _____
Is there anything I should know to ensure your comfort regarding: _____
Allergies/sensitivities: __ oils __ lotions __ scents __ detergents __ foods __ animals __ other: _____
Contact lenses (the face pillow may put pressure on your eyes): _____
Hearing abilities (communication is helpful during the session): _____
Hair, make-up, clothes (Will you return to work after your session?): _____
Movement abilities (i.e., getting on and off the table, pillows, etc.): _____
Comments: _____

Mark on figures all areas of:

Pain, tenderness with O's
Numbness, tingling with ZZ's
Swelling, stiffness with X's
Scars, bruises, open wounds with HH's

Rate severity of all symptom areas from 1-10:

(1 = I feel like a newborn baby, 10 = Put me out of my misery)

1   2   3   4   5   6   7   8   9   10

Previous History

(list in chronological order, give dates or ages, and treatment received)
Surgeries: _____
Accidents: _____
Major illnesses: _____

Consent for Care

It is my choice to receive massage therapy. I am aware of the benefits and risks of massage and give my consent for massage. I understand that there is no implied or stated guarantee of success or effectiveness of individual techniques or series of appointments. I acknowledge that massage therapy is not a substitute for medical care, medical examination, or diagnosis. I have stated all medical conditions that I am aware of and will inform my practitioner of any changes in my health status.

Signature _____ Date _____

© 1999 American Massage Therapy Association, Evanston, Il. All Rights Reserved.

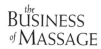

© 2002 American Massage Therapy Association, Evanston, IL. *The Business of Massage.* All Rights Reserved. #20026

Insurance Information

Client's full name _____ Date _____ Ins. ID # _____ DOI _____

Is your condition the result of an auto accident? ___Yes ___No If so, in what state did the accident occur? _____

___ A work injury? ___ A health condition? Other: _____

What type of insurance do you have that may cover you for this condition? (check all that apply)

___ Auto ___ Workers' compensation/State industrial ___ Liability ___ Health

Was a police/accident report filed? ___Yes ___No

Client's relation to insured? Self / Spouse / Partner / Child / Other (circle)

Insured's full name _____ Ins. ID # _____

Date of birth _____ Male / Female   Single / Married / Partnered / Other (circle)

Address _____ City _____ State _____ Zip _____

Phone-Home _____ Work _____ Cell/Pgr _____

Employer's name/school name _____

Address _____ Phone _____

Primary insurance plan name _____

Group number _____ Plan number _____ Phone _____

Plan's billing address _____ City _____ State _____ Zip _____

Secondary insurance information: _____

Who is your attending physician?   Name _____

Address _____ City _____ State _____ Zip _____

Office phone _____ Fax _____

Permission to consult with _____ regarding _____ Your initials _____

Has an attorney been retained? ___Yes ___No Name _____

Address _____ City _____ State _____ Zip _____

Phone-Home _____ Work _____ Fax _____

Assignment of Benefits

I am responsible for all charges for all services provided. In the unfortunate event that my insurance company denies payment, or makes a partial payment, I am responsible for any balance due. If you, my massage therapist, have contracted with my insurance company at a discount rate for services, the amount remaining will be waived and I will not be asked to pay the balance.

I authorize and direct payment of medical benefits to my massage therapist, _____, for services billed.

Signature _____ Date _____

Signature of parent or legal guardian (if client is a minor)

Release of Medical Records

I authorize the release of my medical records or other health care information, including intake forms, chart notes, reports, correspondence, billing statements, and other written information to my attorneys, healthcare providers, and insurance case managers, for the purposes of processing my claims.

Signature _____ Date _____

Signature of parent or legal guardian (if client is a minor)

(Please inform your practitioner immediately upon signing any exclusive Release of Medical Records with your attorney that may impact the above release statement.)

Contract for Care

I will participate fully as a member of my healthcare team. I will make sound choices regarding my sessions' plan based upon the information provided by my massage therapist. I agree to participate in my own self-care program and adhere to the plan we select. I agree to communicate with my practitioner any time I feel my well-being is being compromised. I expect my practitioner to provide safe and effective treatment to the best of his or her skill and knowledge.

Signature _____ Date _____

Signature of parent or legal guardian (if client is a minor)

©1999 American Massage Therapy Association, Evanston, Il. All Rights Reserved.

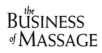

© 2002 American Massage Therapy Association, Evanston, IL. *The Business of Massage.* All Rights Reserved. #20026

Figure 3.16   INFORMED CONSENT SIMPLIFIED FORM

Client Agreement

I, _____, understand that the massage therapy given to me by _____ is for the purposes of stress reduction, pain reduction, relief from muscle tension, increasing circulation, or specific reasons noted here:

I understand that massage therapy does not diagnose illness or disease, or any other disorder, and that the massage therapist does not prescribe medical treatment or pharmaceuticals, nor are spinal manipulations part of massage therapy.

I understand that massage therapy is not a substitute for medical examinations or medical care, and that it is recommended that I am concurrently working with my primary caregiver for any condition I may have.

I have stated all my known physical conditions, medical conditions, and medications, and I will keep the massage therapist updated on any changes.

_____   _____
Client signature   Date

Source: Diane Polseno. "Informed Consent." MASSAGE THERAPY JOURNAL®, Spring 2001. Used with permission.

the
BUSINESS
of MASSAGE

© 2002 American Massage Therapy Association, Evanston, IL. *The Business of Massage.* All Rights Reserved. #20026

Figure 3.17

Request made to:

Name of Massage Practice: _____

Address: _____

City/State/Province _____

Zip/Postal Code: _____

License #: _____

I authorize the release of my medical records or other healthcare information, including intake forms, chart notes, reports, correspondence, billing statements, and other written information to the following person or business:

Name of business/clinician: _____

Address: _____

City/State/Province _____

Zip/Postal Code: _____

Telephone/Fax: _____

E-mail: _____

Client signature: _____ Date: _____

Client name: _____

Date of birth: _____

Social Security Number: _____

If this authorization should cover more than a single release of information, please specify dates below:

Authorization is valid until: _____ (date).

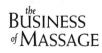

© 2002 American Massage Therapy Association, Evanston, IL. *The Business of Massage.* All Rights Reserved. #20026

Shared Wisdom

"Chart every single session, regardless of the intent of the session (relaxation or rehabilitation), regardless of the payor (cash or insurance), and regardless of the health of the client. The chart entry can be as simple as: '2-2-03, full body Swedish massage, client prefers pillow under hips when prone,' or as complex as a SOAP chart. If we are to be treated as healthcare providers, we are to behave as such. Think of it this way— a doctor would never consider skipping out on charting an annual physical just because the patient is in good health."

—Diana Thompson, author of Hands Heal: Communication, Documentation, and Insurance Billing for Manual Therapists

SOAP Notes

You will also need a consistent, objective way to keep records of clients' needs and the work provided in each session, while demonstrating the client's progress. While used in many settings, SOAP notes are the most common method for charting a patient's health problems and care in hospital and medical settings. SOAP notes (for Subjective, Objective, Assessment, Plan) provide the following benefits:

1. Increased ability to understand patients' care and progress when reviewing patients' medical charts
2. Increased ability to succinctly communicate practitioner's care services and their results for your future reference
3. Increased ability to communicate care services and results to other medical staff
4. Improved likelihood of insurance reimbursement
5. Through demonstration of the above, increased respect from medical staff

Adapted from "Writing SOAP Notes," by Ginge Kettenbach, reviewed by Laura Koch in *The Hospital-Based Massage Network Quarterly*, Fall 1998, Vol. 4, No. 3.

This format has four parts:

1. The client's subjective complaints and functional goals, including symptoms, affected daily activities, and the client's goals for the session (e.g., "mild shoulder pain, increases with lifting; goal: to lift child without pain")
2. The massage practitioner's objective findings and recommended plan ("tender point—right trapezius, mild right shoulder elevation, direct pressure with active assisted movement")
3. The massage practitioner's assessment (to demonstrate progress)—rating the client's subjective changes and the massage therapist's objective changes as a result of the session(s) (e.g., "no shoulder pain; right shoulder elevation within normal limits") Note that diagnosis or prognosis is not within the scope of practice for massage therapists.
4. The massage therapist's plan for future care and the client's self-care plan, coordinating the session frequency with a doctor's prescription as necessary (e.g., "weekly massage to reduce shoulder pain; ice shoulder 8 to 10 minutes as needed")

Gathering this much information on healthy clients might be difficult. Not all clients receive massage therapy to address physical ailments. "Soap Charts" (figure 3.18, page 147) show two methods of SOAP charting to record information specific to the needs of relaxation and medical massage. [Source: "Manual Three: Managing Your Practice," *AMTA Massage Therapy Career Guide.* American Massage Therapy Association, 1999, pages 26-27.]

Client Telephone Log

Another form that is useful as a client record is a form for telephone follow-up. You can build ongoing, beneficial relationships with clients by calling them the day after a session to check how they are feeling. When you call, take notes on what you learn.

Client Visits and Billing Record

Keep a running client log by date. This record of client visits should include patient name, session type and duration, total charges and adjustments, payment amount, and any amount to be billed to an insurance company. See "Record of Client Visits" (figure 3.19, page 148).

Figure 3.18

SOAP CHARTS

SOAP FOR RELAXATION MASSAGE

Client Name _____

Session Type _____ Duration _____ Date _____

S: Goals for Session

O: Techniques Applied

A: Comments

P: Follow-up

Provider Initials _____

SOAP FOR MEDICAL MASSAGE

Client Name _____ Date _____

Insurance ID number _____ Date of Injury _____

Modality Type (code) _____ Duration _____

Modality Type (code) _____ Duration _____

Current Medications _____

S: Functional Goals

   Symptoms: Location/Intensity/Duration/Frequency/Onset

   Activities Affected by Condition

O: Visual/Palpable Findings, Modalities

A: Resulting Subjective and Objective Changes

P: Massage Plan/Self Care Homework

✕ Adhesion	• Tender Point	⚡ Inflammation
⟲ Rotation	≡ Hypertonicity	◎ Trigger Point
○ Pain	≈ Spasm	╱ Elevation

Provider Initials _____

©1999 American Massage Therapy Association, Evanston, Il. All Rights Reserved.

the
BUSINESS
of MASSAGE

© 2002 American Massage Therapy Association, Evanston, IL. *The Business of Massage.* All Rights Reserved. #20026

Figure 3.19

RECORD OF CLIENT VISITS

Week of _____

Date	Name	Session Type	Duration	Total Charges	Adjustments	Payments	Insurance to Be Billed
Mon	Jim Smith	Relax	30 min.	$35.00	10% cash discount	$31.50	——
Mon	Sally Jones	Med.	60 min.	$60.00	——	$15 co-pay	$45

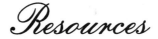

Resources

Information and Forms for Client Documentation

- AMTA. *The Business of Massage Business Forms Packet.* Evanston, IL: American Massage Therapy Association, 2002.
- Ashley, Martin. *A Career at Your Fingertips, Third Edition.* Carmel, NY: Enterprise Publishing, 1999.
- Bates, Barbara, Lynn S. Bickley, Robert A. Hoekelman. *A Pocket Guide to Bates' Physical Examination and History Taking.* Philadelphia: Lippincott Williams & Wilkins, 1999.
- Kettenbach, Ginge. *Writing SOAP Notes.* Philadelphia, PA: F.A. Davis Company, 1995.
- Medical Arts Press: 8500 Wyoming Ave. N., Minneapolis, MN 55445; 800-328-2179; www.medicalartspress.com
- Persad, Randal S. *Massage Therapy Medications.* Toronto: Curties-Overzet Publications Inc., 2001; 1-888-649-5411
- Saunders, Jefferson C. *Your Successful Massage/Bodywork Practice, Revised Third Edition.* Seattle: Superior Publishing, Inc., 1995).
- Sohnen-Moe, Cherie. *Business Mastery, Third Edition.* Phoenix: Sohnen-Moe Associates, Inc., 1997.
- Thompson, Diana L. *Hands Heal: Communication, Documentation, and Insurance Billing for Manual Therapists.* Lippincott Williams & Wilkins, 2001.
- Walton, Tracy. "Taking a Health History." *Massage Therapy Journal,* Winter 1999.

Administrative Management

Insurance

As a massage practitioner, you will need to decide whether to accept clients whose massages are paid for by insurance (also known as third-party reimbursement). This section will help you make that decision. (For information about your own insurance needs as a practitioner, see the section "Insurance—Protecting Yourself from Loss" in chapter 2, pages 92-95.)

Client Insurance

You may have the opportunity to provide services covered by some form of insurance. Nearly 20 percent of AMTA members collect insurance reimbursement for their client work, and another nearly 30 percent are interested in participating in this type of reimbursement [AMTA 2000 Segmentation Survey].

Over the past several years massage therapy has made great progress in being accepted as a healthcare service covered by some insurance programs. There are three types of such insurance, and multiple categories for each of these types, that may cover massage therapy:
1. Auto insurance
2. Workers' compensation
3. Health insurance

Knowing the intent of each type of coverage will help you know when to expect payment from an insurance company or client. According to AMTA, the most common forms of third-party reimbursement are from automobile insurance (20 percent), health insurance (17 percent), and workers' compensation insurance (13 percent).

In order for massage therapy to qualify for third-party reimbursements, the service must be prescribed by a physician, and the massage service must be delivered under supervision of the prescribing doctor. Insurance companies have final decision authority on all third-party reimbursements.

Many insurance companies offer alternative approaches through which to respond to consumer demand for massage. Some companies offer alternative/complementary benefits, for which the subscriber (your client) pays a premium, just as an individual would pay for any type of health insurance coverage. The number of massages, or other alternative health services, a subscriber may receive depends on the type of benefit he or she purchased.

Another approach to alternative/complementary programs that insurance companies use is discount programs, often called affinity plans. For massage practitioners to participate in either of these types of programs, they must agree to discount their fees, often about 25 percent off the practitioner's usual fee. For more information, see section on "Client Health Insurance" on page 155.

Depending on where you live and what the reimbursement climate is like, a massage practitioner should balance income from third-party reimbursement clients and out-of-pocket payers. Some practitioners feel it is smart to collect about half of their income from out-of-pocket clients in order to balance their cash flow.

Be aware that seeking third-party reimbursement clients and collaborating with the traditional medical establishment is an area some massage practitioners view as controversial. AMTA member surveys indicate a general trend of newer practitioners seeking third-party reimbursement clients to help them establish their clients quickly. Practitioners who do not accept insurance clients say they prefer to be paid on a cash basis, and they want to set their own fees and not wait for payments to be processed. See "Pros and Cons of Seeking Third-Party Reimbursement" (figure 3.20, page 151).

Submitting Claims

Massage practitioners who have experience submitting claims for third-party reimbursement offer the following advice for successful and timely receipt of payment:

- Attach the patient's prescription to the claim, indicating that massage services are medically necessary. The prescription should contain the patient's diagnosis, specify that massage is the prescribed service, and the location, frequency, and duration of the sessions.
- If the massage practitioner works in a doctor's office, ask that the office process the claim.
- Contact the claims representative or insurance adjuster in advance of the claim being filed. The individual who will process the claim may have misunderstandings about massage, and it can be helpful if the massage therapist speaks directly with the underwriter to ask questions such as, "What specifically do you want me to provide?" (This could be a copy of your license, a copy of the prescription, a copy of the session notes, or progress reports.)
- Include the appropriate CPT (Common Procedural Terminology) codes. CPT codes are used only by licensed healthcare providers, and as such they identify the healthcare service being provided. (See this chapter's section on "Billing Insurance Companies," page 159, for a disclaimer about using CPT codes.)
- Because CPT codes change, be sure to verify the code in a CPT manual before using it.

Figure 3.20: Pros and Cons of Seeking Third-Party Reimbursement

Pros

Insurance coverage provides access to a potentially large and growing client base.

Insurance plans may be willing to pay more than individuals in the area.

More people will be apt to receive massage if it is a covered benefit.

If you work through or for hospitals and clinics, they might handle or help with billing.

You could use insurance clients to supplement your self-paid client base.

Working for an HMO or clinic, you could have a steady flow of income.

You are educating the providers and insurance carriers about the benefits of massage.

The insurance company may advertise your practice.

Your referral base is from other respected healthcare professionals.

Cons

You would have to work within the insurance company's system.

You will have to do a lot of paperwork, including maintaining SOAP notes and filing claims.

The insurance company or referring doctor may define the type and extent of care you provide.

You may have to meet insurance plan requirements such as number of minutes allowed per session or number of sessions for a particular condition.

Your contract with an insurance company may prohibit you from accepting cash payments over the amount the insurance company will pay.

Your fee may be limited by the plan coverage, and payment may be slow or even denied.

You may experience lengthy delays in receiving payments.

Source: American Massage Therapy Association. *Health Insurance Reimbursement Facts.* 1999.

For more information about the pros and cons of insurance reimbursement for massage practitioners, see "Insurance Reimbursement: Pros and Cons," by David Munsey (pro) and David M. Frederick (con). *Massage Therapy Journal*, Summer 2001, pages 40-47.

Auto Insurance

Clients may have coverage for massage therapy as part of their auto insurance policy, or benefits. For example, someone injured in a car accident may be covered for massage treatments as part of the insurance policy. If you agree to take this client, you may need to arrange payment from the insurance company, rather than from the injured person. There are different levels of medical coverage through auto insurance:

- *First party*—The client is covered by the benefits in the client's own auto policy, called Personal Injury Protection (PIP) coverage. First-party coverage usually pays the massage therapist for care while the case is ongoing. The therapist should contact the insurance company to verify that the client has benefits and has not exhausted the amount of coverage purchased. If the client has used up all the coverage for medical payments, then the company is not required to pay the service provider. Payment for care becomes part of a possible settlement, but the insurance company has no obligation to pay for those massage sessions.

- *Third party*—The client is covered by the insurance of another person (the at-fault party). In this situation, the massage therapist treating the client may either receive payment from the insurance company at the end of the case (settlement), or the therapist may be paid by the client, who pays directly and then submits the bills to the insurance company at the end of the case. In the latter situation, the therapist receives payment while providing care, and the client is reimbursed at settlement. The massage therapist must provide clear invoices for the care given. It is helpful to use standard billing receipts, or billing forms, such as "HCFA 1500 Billing Form" (figure 3.21, page 153). HCFA has been renamed Centers for Medicare and Medicaid Services, CMMS. Some states require that you submit these forms electronically rather than hard copy.

For both first-party and third-party coverage of medical injuries in an auto accident, the care usually requires a physician's prescription or written referral. (See "Referral Form from Physician," figure 3.22, page 154). The care must be medically necessary, and fees should be reasonable.

Smoothing Your Way with Auto Insurance

- Make good chart notes and document the type of care you provide in each session. Be prepared to provide copies of SOAP notes to the insurance company and/or attorneys working on the case.
- Work on the specific areas of injury as well as the surrounding areas, and, when asked for a report on the client's progress, do not diagnose or offer a prognosis. Only indicate in writing the changes you see.
- Keep your fees reasonable for the market in which you are practicing. If your fees are substantially higher than those of other therapists in your area, the insurance company may pay you a reduced rate.
- Be sure to have your client sign an agreement that if PIP (personal injury protection) insurance limits are reached or care is denied, the client is responsible for the cost of the care.

Figure 3.21

PLEASE
DO NOT
STAPLE
IN THIS
AREA

APPROVED OMB-0938-0008

CARRIER

HEALTH INSURANCE CLAIM FORM

PICA | | PICA

1. MEDICARE (Medicare #) MEDICAID (Medicaid #) CHAMPUS (Sponsor s SSN) CHAMPVA (VA File #) GROUP HEALTH PLAN (SSN or ID) FECA BLK LUNG (SSN) OTHER (ID) | 1a. INSURED S I.D. NUMBER (FOR PROGRAM IN ITEM 1)

2. PATIENT S NAME (Last Name, First Name, Middle Initial)

3. PATIENT S BIRTH DATE MM DD YY SEX M F

4. INSURED S NAME (Last Name, First Name, Middle Initial)

5. PATIENT S ADDRESS (No., Street)

6. PATIENT RELATIONSHIP TO INSURED Self Spouse Child Other

7. INSURED S ADDRESS (No., Street)

CITY STATE

8. PATIENT STATUS Single Married Other
Employed Full-Time Student Part-Time Student

CITY STATE

ZIP CODE TELEPHONE (Include Area Code) ( )

ZIP CODE TELEPHONE (INCLUDE AREA CODE) ( )

9. OTHER INSURED S NAME (Last Name, First Name, Middle Initial)

10. IS PATIENT S CONDITION RELATED TO:

11. INSURED S POLICY GROUP OR FECA NUMBER

a. OTHER INSURED S POLICY OR GROUP NUMBER

a. EMPLOYMENT? (CURRENT OR PREVIOUS) YES NO

a. INSURED S DATE OF BIRTH MM DD YY SEX M F

b. OTHER INSURED S DATE OF BIRTH MM DD YY SEX M F

b. AUTO ACCIDENT? PLACE (State) YES NO

b. EMPLOYER S NAME OR SCHOOL NAME

c. EMPLOYER S NAME OR SCHOOL NAME

c. OTHER ACCIDENT? YES NO

c. INSURANCE PLAN NAME OR PROGRAM NAME

d. INSURANCE PLAN NAME OR PROGRAM NAME

10d. RESERVED FOR LOCAL USE

d. IS THERE ANOTHER HEALTH BENEFIT PLAN? YES NO *If yes,* return to and complete item 9 a-d.

READ BACK OF FORM BEFORE COMPLETING & SIGNING THIS FORM.

12. PATIENT S OR AUTHORIZED PERSON S SIGNATURE I authorize the release of any medical or other information necessary to process this claim. I also request payment of government benefits either to myself or to the party who accepts assignment below.

SIGNED _____ DATE _____

13. INSURED S OR AUTHORIZED PERSON S SIGNATURE I authorize payment of medical benefits to the undersigned physician or supplier for services described below.

SIGNED _____

PATIENT AND INSURED INFORMATION

14. DATE OF CURRENT: MM DD YY ILLNESS (First symptom) OR INJURY (Accident) OR PREGNANCY(LMP)

15. IF PATIENT HAS HAD SAME OR SIMILAR ILLNESS. GIVE FIRST DATE MM DD YY

16. DATES PATIENT UNABLE TO WORK IN CURRENT OCCUPATION FROM MM DD YY TO MM DD YY

17. NAME OF REFERRING PHYSICIAN OR OTHER SOURCE

17a. I.D. NUMBER OF REFERRING PHYSICIAN

18. HOSPITALIZATION DATES RELATED TO CURRENT SERVICES FROM MM DD YY TO MM DD YY

19. RESERVED FOR LOCAL USE

20. OUTSIDE LAB? YES NO $ CHARGES

21. DIAGNOSIS OR NATURE OF ILLNESS OR INJURY. (RELATE ITEMS 1,2,3 OR 4 TO ITEM 24E BY LINE)
1. ____.__   3. ____.__
2. ____.__   4. ____.__

22. MEDICAID RESUBMISSION CODE ORIGINAL REF. NO.

23. PRIOR AUTHORIZATION NUMBER

24. A DATE(S) OF SERVICE						B Place of Service	C Type of Service	D PROCEDURES, SERVICES, OR SUPPLIES (Explain Unusual Circumstances) CPT/HCPCS MODIFIER	E DIAGNOSIS CODE	F $ CHARGES	G DAYS OR UNITS	H EPSDT Family Plan	I EMG	J COB	K RESERVED FOR LOCAL USE
From MM	DD	YY	To MM	DD	YY										
1															
2															
3															
4															
5															
6															

25. FEDERAL TAX I.D. NUMBER SSN EIN

26. PATIENT S ACCOUNT NO.

27. ACCEPT ASSIGNMENT? (For govt. claims, see back) YES NO

28. TOTAL CHARGE $

29. AMOUNT PAID $

30. BALANCE DUE $

31. SIGNATURE OF PHYSICIAN OR SUPPLIER INCLUDING DEGREES OR CREDENTIALS (I certify that the statements on the reverse apply to this bill and are made a part thereof.)

SIGNED _____ DATE _____

32. NAME AND ADDRESS OF FACILITY WHERE SERVICES WERE RENDERED (If other than home or office)

33. PHYSICIAN S, SUPPLIER S BILLING NAME, ADDRESS, ZIP CODE & PHONE #

PIN# GRP#

PHYSICIAN OR SUPPLIER INFORMATION

(APPROVED BY AMA COUNCIL ON MEDICAL SERVICE 8/88) **PLEASE PRINT OR TYPE** FORM HCFA-1500 (12-90), FORM RRB-1500, FORM OWCP-1500

the BUSINESS *of* MASSAGE

© 2002 American Massage Therapy Association, Evanston, IL. *The Business of Massage.* All Rights Reserved. #20026

Figure 3.22

Patient Name _____ Ins. ID # _____ Date of Injury _____ Date _____
Diagnosis (include ICD-9 codes specifically addressing massage therapy care): _____
_____
_____

Direct and Indirect Areas of Concern:
__ cervical __ thoracic __ lumbar/lumbosacral
__ cranial __ scapular __ upper extremities
__ lower extremities __ other:

Precautions: _____
_____

Condition is Related to: ❏ auto accident ❏ work injury ❏ general medical ❏ other: _____

Care Plan:
Rx Frequency: ❏ 1x/wk ❏ 2x/wk ❏ 3x/wk ❏ 1x/2wks ❏ 1x/4wks for _____ weeks.

Care Type:
❏ massage ❏ hydrotherapy ❏ self care education

Specific Instructions: _____
_____

Care Goals:
__ increase mobility __ increase strength __ restore function __ restore posture
__ decrease pain __ decrease inflammation __ decrease muscle tension/spasms
__ decrease compensational adaptation syndrome __ maintain associated structures

Additional Comments: _____
_____
_____
_____
_____

__ Send report after initial visit.
__ Send report at end of prescription.
__ Send copies of chart notes at end of prescription.
__ Fax information __ Mail information __ Call with information __ E-mail information

Physician's Signature _____ Date _____

Physician Name: _____
Address: _____
City/State/Zip: _____
Telephone: _____ E-mail: _____ Fax: _____

the BUSINESS *of* MASSAGE

© 2002 American Massage Therapy Association, Evanston, IL. *The Business of Massage.* All Rights Reserved. #20026

Workers' Compensation

Workers' compensation is the benefit that covers an employee injured while at work. The claim that an injured worker files must be approved before payment of any claims to a healthcare provider. Usually a doctor must refer the client for massage therapy, and the referral usually outlines the length of time that the care is approved. Some states require that a provider not take any money from a client unless and until the claim is denied. At the time a claim is denied, the client becomes responsible for all costs incurred with the provider.

The focus of workers' compensation is to return the client to work. This requires that the service provider take notes that mention objective data related to the client's job activities. Be sure to use SOAP notes and to keep your work in accordance with the referring provider's orders.

Client Health Insurance

Health insurance coverage for massage therapy has increased dramatically in the past several years. Insurance companies are practicing multiple methods of coverage and establishing different rules that the provider must follow or else be declared ineligible to receive reimbursement. However, many insurance companies do not cover massage therapy at all or, if they do, cover it under the physical medicine code, which usually is quite limited. When massage therapy is covered, often there are rules as to which provider category may perform the massage. In most cases, health insurance companies cover massage only when the massage is provided by a physician, chiropractor, or physical therapist. This is changing slowly, but many insurance companies have not yet decided to cover massage therapy by a massage therapist.

When massage is covered, different types of coverage are available:
* The insurance company may offer its members, or enrollees, access to a list of providers that agree to accept a discounted rate. To be on the list, therapists usually must sign a contract. As part of the contract, the insurance company sets the fee, and the therapist may not charge the client more than the agreed-upon fee. The contract may have additional requirements as well—for example, that therapists must work in a professional setting (not in their homes), carry a specified level of professional liability insurance, and be licensed or, where there is no state license, have practiced massage for a period of time. (Especially in states that do not regulate massage therapists, it is beneficial to have National Certification for Therapeutic Massage and Bodywork.) In exchange for these requirements, the insurance company promises to market the massage therapist's name to its enrollees. As with any contract, you should read the contract with a health insurance company carefully before signing it. If in doubt, have an attorney review it.
* Some insurance companies offer a wellness benefit. Companies that buy this benefit offer their members access to massage therapists who are preferred providers. The insurance company may even offer coverage for massage therapists under the policy's general medical coverage, but with limitations. These providers are referred to as "in-network" providers. Contracts with preferred providers usually have more requirements than those that merely offer a discounted rate. The providers must have professional liability insurance with specified amounts of coverage. (The standard is $1 million per occurrence with a $3 million annual

aggregate.) The provider must accept the fee the insurance company pays, and clients must be referred for services by their primary care provider (PCP). Usually, the insurance company limits the conditions that the massage therapist may bill for; the type of massage technique may also be limited. Finally, the contract with preferred providers usually requires that they must have been in practice for at least a specified period of time and must work in a professional setting rather than a residence.

The most significant difference between the two types of contracts is that preferred providers must be willing to accept any client who is covered by the plan. You may not "balance bill" the client, charging any difference between what you normally charge and what the insurance company will reimburse. Most important, these contracts frequently contain clauses (sometimes in accordance with laws) stating that if the insurance company goes out of business, you may not charge any unpaid balances to the client receiving the care. This type of clause, called a "hold harmless" clause, is prevalent in many contracts with providers (including doctors and nurses). In exchange for this, the insurance company promises to market your practice to its members.

Working with Healthcare Providers

If, after reviewing the issues made in "Pros and Cons of Seeking Third-Party Reimbursement" (figure 3.20, page 151), you are interested in working with insurance companies, it is important to establish how your care will address your clients' particular problems. You will probably need to work with healthcare providers; they will make medical diagnoses and refer clients to you. "Healthcare Providers with Whom AMTA Members Work" (figure 3.23, page 157) shows the extent to which AMTA members who practice full-time and part-time work with various types of healthcare professionals. Note that those who work with healthcare professionals have significantly higher incomes.

If you would like to work with healthcare providers, you will have to build professional relationships with them. Brief guidelines about how to become approved as a healthcare provider by insurance companies are included here. See chapter 7 for more information on building professional networks.

Building Relationships with Healthcare Providers

- Be sure you have adequate training in the modalities that are appropriate for injuries or diseases that healthcare practitioners work with, including neuromuscular therapy (NMT), myofascial therapy, manual lymph drainage (MLD), and deep tissue massage. If your entry-level education did not provide enough of this training, look for relevant courses at massage schools, community colleges, or at other continuing education sources. See chapter 8 for a list of resources for continuing education.
- Send allied healthcare practitioners a letter that speaks in medical terms, such as "Sample Introduction Letter to Healthcare Practitioners" (figure 3.24, page 158). Show them that you have a working knowledge of anatomy and physiology and that you understand how the medical community handles patients. Healthcare providers who refer patients to massage therapists may include chiropractors, rheumatologists, internists, neurologists, doctors of family medicine, obstetricians and gynecologists, doctors of sports medicine, physical therapists, and psychiatrists.

- Follow up with the healthcare providers. Make an appointment during their off-business hours, because they are most likely to be available then. For example, you could meet ten minutes before or after they have lunch. See "Healthcare Provider Follow-up Outline" (figure 3.25, page 159).
- Provide qualifications, including a summary of your education and experience. If your state requires licensure, show that you are licensed in the state and/or are Nationally Certified and/or are a member of a well-respected professional association.
- Have data that support the efficacy of massage. You can get such data from AMTA's Web site in the Massage Information Center section.
- Tell healthcare providers why you should work together.
- Explain how you will measure the success of your work. David Dolan, of Advanced Therapeutics America, P.A., uses postural analysis, on the theory that postural balance is associated with reduction of symptoms. Dolan told *Massage Therapy Journal* that this provides the kind of objective measure that is helpful in communicating with physicians and insurance companies. Other possible measurements include an analog pain scale, the Revised Oswestry Questionnaire, the Vernon Mior questionnaire, trigger points charting, and, if trained to do so, the range of motion of affected muscle groups. These forms/charts can be found at medical or massage supply outlets. Training in certain therapies, including NMT and MLD, should cover charting methods.
- Explain your process of working with clients. Include procedures such as client intake (noting prescription), charting (on SOAP notes), exit interview with client (on SOAP notes), follow-up form to healthcare provider (sent after one to two visits) in which you state the care provided and progress the client is making. Illustrate your explanation with examples of forms on which you have "whited out" the names of the clients, to protect confidentiality.
- Demonstrate your competence. You may decide to enhance your credibility by providing the healthcare provider, office manager, or nurse with a complimentary massage, demonstrating what you do, how you do it, and why you do it. The combination of sample forms and a sample massage are a great way to demonstrate your professionalism and skill. You also show you are able to communicate with healthcare providers in a common language.

Source: Mary Anne Fleetwood. "A Program to Get Those Elusive Insurance Reimbursement Dollars." *Massage Therapy Journal*, Spring/Summer 1997, pages 93-94, 96, 98.

Figure 3.23: Healthcare Providers with Whom AMTA Members Work

Type of Provider	Full-time Massage Therapists	Part-time Massage Therapists
Chiropractors	67%	51%
Medical doctors	56%	38%
Physical therapists	40%	25%
Nurse/nurse practitioners	33%	21%
Psychotherapists/psychologists	9%	6%

Source: American Massage Therapy Association Segmentation Study 2000. Used by permission.

Figure 3.24

SAMPLE INTRODUCTION LETTER
to Healthcare Practitioners

ABC MASSAGE THERAPY, INC.
123 Any Street
Anywhere, USA
(555) 555-5555

(Date)

Dear Dr._____:

My name is (Diane Taylor) and I am a (licensed) massage therapist. (I am new in your area/We are sharing a patient for the first time) and I wanted to tell you a little bit about myself and the kind of work that I do, (in the event that we may work together in the future). It is my intention to support your healthcare plan and to provide quality care to your patients.

I have experience in actively participating on healthcare teams and am able to communicate through standard forms of documentation. Enclosed are sample copies of my charting and report writing style. I am committed to keeping my referring physicians apprised of their patients' progress.

My specialty is (headaches). I have attended advanced study courses on this condition and have taken a special interest in (headaches relating to whiplash trauma.) I am also highly skilled in (the treatment of a variety of musculoskeletal dysfunctions). Enclosed are copies of my educational certificates (and license/National Certification credentials).

The massage modalities I utilize most often include (trigger point therapy and manual lymphatic drainage). My clinic is well equipped to provide state-of-the-art (hydrotherapy) treatment.

I have enclosed brochures on my clinic, detailing my services, the hours I am available, and the fees for the various treatment options. I have included brochures illustrating the benefits of massage therapy and the specifics of (manual lymph drainage). Additionally, I am including my Code of Ethics and Standards of Practice and my professional association membership certificate.

Professionalism, communication, and quality health care are my strengths. Please share my brochures and call me if you or your patients have the need for an exceptional massage therapist.

I look forward to working with you in the future.

Yours in health,

(name)
Licensed Massage Therapist, NCTMB

Encl.:   Code of Ethics
         Standards of Practice
         Professional association membership certificate
         Brochures

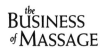

© 2002 American Massage Therapy Association, Evanston, IL. *The Business of Massage.* All Rights Reserved.   #20026

Figure 3.25: Healthcare Provider Follow-up Outline

When communicating with healthcare professionals, sometimes the quality of communicating is higher if you write a letter or report rather than use a form. When you provide follow-up status on a client's care to a physician, the following information should be included in your letter or report:
- Restatement of goals for client's care
- Description of care provided and client's progress
- Projected goals if client care is extended to more visits

Billing Insurance Companies

When you are seeking third-party reimbursement, you must bill the insurance company according to its requirements. For example, Medicare denies claims submitted more than eighteen months after the service was provided, and some health maintenance organizations (HMOs) and Preferred Provider Organizations (PPOs) deny payment for claims submitted after a specific time frame, such as sixty to ninety days after services were provided. To avoid losing the entire payment, it is essential to submit claims within such deadlines.

Insurers need to keep detailed records on a wide variety of clients and situations, so they create precise systems for recording that information. Before you provide a massage to a client who may be covered by insurance, contact the client's insurance company and ask for billing instructions. If you can bill electronically, this may be faster and less expensive. Also ask whether the company requires you to fill out a form to be accepted as a provider. If possible, have the company send you written authorization to perform the services. In some cases, prior authorization is required for reimbursement. Unfortunately, however, preapproval does not guarantee payment from an insurance company.

Be sure to note the date and time of each call to the insurance company, along with the name of the person with whom you spoke and what was said. File these notes in an A-to-Z "Billed but Not Collected" file under the client's name. That way, it is easy to follow up if you do not receive payment within thirty days.

You may need to use specific names and codes for the client's conditions and the modalities provided in the session. The insurance company will tell you what Current Procedural Terminology (CPT) code to use, but you must meet the company's qualifications for care. (Understand your state's regulations regarding CPT codes. In New York, for example, massage therapists do not use CPTs.) Or, if you are part of a complementary/alternative medicine discount plan, that plan may have its own coding system. Note that only doctors are permitted to diagnose, so any diagnostic codes must come from the office of the doctor who referred the client. Ideally, these codes should be stated on a prescription pad. Also, if you are in a state that does not regulate massage therapists, you may not be able to do your own billing; you may have to work through a doctor's office.

Shared Wisdom

"A massage therapist must find common ground with the medical community in their communication of what it is they do and how long it will take. When a massage therapist starts talking energy and meridians, the doctor's eyes will glaze over. Tell them what you can do for their patient in anatomical and physiological terms and your specific care plan for a given medical condition. Help them feel comfortable that referring a patient to you was the right thing to do."

—Bob Haase,
Bodymechanics School of
Myotherapy & Massage,
Olympia, Washington

Tips on Billing Insurance Companies

1. The physician's order for your client's treatment should include: the diagnosis code or codes, the frequency of treatments, total number of treatments, doctor's name and identification number (UPIN), and a statement that massage is medically necessary.

2. Once the client contacts you, you need to confirm coverage for your services. Ask your client for: name, date of birth, Social Security number, address, phone numbers, date of injury, insurance company name, policy number, and name of insured party.

3. Contact the client's insurance company. Tell the receptionist you are calling for pre-approval. When you reach the appropriate department, write down the name of the person you speak with and ask how to contact him or her in the future. Explain that you are a massage therapist, that massage has been declared "medically necessary" by the insured's physician, and that you are seeking pre-approval for your services.

4. Depending on the type of work you do, and the company you are dealing with, you may wish to describe your services as "soft-tissue mobilization," "myofascial release," or "massage therapy."

5. Find out from the insurance representative: 1) how many visits will be paid for; 2) how much the company will pay per visit; 3) what CPT code procedures are acceptable; and 4) whether there are any restrictions on who performs the services or where the services are performed.

6. Get a written release from your client that gives you permission to submit bills and SOAP notes to the insurance company.

7. Perform the hands-on treatment. Do SOAP charting.

8. As client care progresses, submit bills for your services to the insurance company. Use what is called the superbill, or HCFA 1500. Be sure you understand the difference between a diagnostic code and a CPT code. (See reference books for more detail.)

9. If you have not received payment in 45 days, follow up with a phone call to the individual you spoke with initially at the insurance company. Make sure your bill was received, and find out if there is any reason it has not been paid.

Adapted from "Business Wise," by Martin Ashley. *Massage Magazine*, January/February 2000, pages 70, 75-78.

Insurance Paperwork

When a client is covered by insurance, be especially careful with your paperwork. Keep copies of the following documents in the client's folder:

- the client's insurance card(s)—copies of front and back
- the prescription and/or other referral document from the client's doctor
- the insurance preapproval request
- for workers' compensation, the Statement of Injury form
- an authorization, signed by the client, for you to release medical information (Some states set time limits on how long the signature is valid.)
- a statement, signed by the client, stating that the client will pay any charges not covered by insurance
- SOAP notes
- the reports used to update the referring healthcare provider

In addition, in a "Billed but Not Collected" file, keep the following forms:
- any claim forms you file with the insurer
- any correspondence, notes of conversations, and forms related to inquiries about or denials of claims
- a log of outstanding insurance claims, as shown in "Client Insurance Log" (figure 3.26, page 162), indicating the name of the client; his or her insurance company; the invoice number, amount, and date billed; and any partial payment and date paid

Whether you decide to accept or not accept third-party reimbursement clients, it is important to be aware of what is required to administer these clients.

Health Insurance Portability and Accountability Act—HIPAA

New government regulations go into effect at the end of February 2003 for providers of healthcare services who file insurance claims electronically. The name of this regulatory document is HIPAA, Health Insurance Portability and Accountability Act. It specifies that if you seek insurance reimbursement for your services as a healthcare provider, and if you use electronic methods in conducting your transactions, HIPAA affects you.

HIPAA is a federal regulation that is intended to simplify the electronic transactions involved in administering and interacting with healthcare plans. The results are intended to streamline the processing of healthcare claims, reduce the volume of paperwork, and provide better service for providers, insurers and patients and, in doing so, to reduce the national costs associated with health care.

If you are a massage practitioner who electronically submits claims to health plans as a service provider, HIPAA means that you need to follow a new set of rules in order to be reimbursed. New rules go into effect in the following areas:

Electronic Transactions

The method of filing claims on-line, or electronically, is known as Electronic Data Interchange (EDI). HIPAA does not mandate the use of EDI, but requires the use of specific standards if EDI is used. If you file electronically, you must comply with the new HIPAA standards. The reason for national standards is to make conducting these transactions simpler and less costly, by establishing a single set of rules that all healthcare plans, providers, and organizations must follow.

The types of EDI transactions for which HIPAA mandates standards for health plans include:
- claims
- enrollment/disenrollment
- eligibility
- payment and remittance advice
- premium payments
- claim status
- referral certification and authorization
- coordination of benefits

Figure 3.26

CLIENT INSURANCE LOG

Client Name _____ Invoice# _____ Date of Injury _____

Insurance Company _____

Amount Billed:

Session Date	Modalities (CPT Codes)	Duration (Units)	Total Charges	Adjustments	Billing Date	Amount Billed
						Total

Amount Paid:

Date of Payment by Client	Total Amount Paid by Client	Date of Payment by Insurance	Total Amount Paid by Insurance
		Total	

Amount Rebilled:

Rebilling Date to Insurance	Added Interest	New Total Billed
		Total

Notes: _____

© 2002 American Massage Therapy Association, Evanston, IL. *The Business of Massage*. All Rights Reserved. #20026

the BUSINESS *of* MASSAGE

If you file electronically but are unable, or do not choose, to comply with HIPAA standards, you have the option of filing through a clearinghouse that will submit your transactions in the compliant format.

One of the possible outcomes of HIPAA is that electronic methodology could become the standard method for transactions of healthcare claims in the future. If you now conduct all transactions manually, this new emphasis on electronic filing might encourage you to increase your knowledge and use of technology in order to stay abreast of industry changes.

National Provider Identifier

Each healthcare provider who conducts transactions electronically will be assigned a National Provider Identifier (NPI). This NPI will be used by all health plans as the number that uniquely identifies you as a service provider. This is a change from the current environment, where providers are assigned a different identification number by multiple health plans. To learn more about NPI, go to www.aspe.hhs.gov/admnsimp/faqnpi.htm.

Privacy of Client Information

HIPAA mandates new security standards to protect an individual's health information, while permitting the appropriate access and use of that information by healthcare providers, clearinghouses and health plans. Protection of client health information, if it is transmitted electronically, is required in order to prevent misuse of any individually identifiable information. Some of the ways in which HIPAA assures these protections include the following:
- Providers are required to give patients a written explanation of how they use, keep, and disclose the patient's health information.
- Patients must be able to see and access copies of their records.
- Providers are required to obtain patient consent before sharing the patient's information electronically, and patients have the right to request restrictions on the uses and disclosures of their information.

You need to learn how HIPAA requirements for security standards might impact the way in which you collect, store, or share client information. For more information, go to www.aspe.hhs.gov/admnsimp/faqsec.htm.

New Codes to Describe Procedures and Impairments

New HIPAA standards for electronic transactions change the procedures and codes you use in communicating with clients, healthcare plans, and other healthcare organizations. You need to learn what the new rules are and the time frames for implementing them.

Penalties for Noncompliance

HIPAA requirements apply to all private sector and government health plans, all healthcare clearinghouses, and all healthcare providers who choose to submit or receive healthcare transactions electronically. Penalties for noncompliance start at $100 for each violation, and up to $25,000 maximum for multiple violations of identical requirements. Penalties for wrongful disclosure of individually identifiable health information can include prison time and fines up to $250,000.

Source: "Massage Therapy and HIPAA: How HIPAA May Affect Massage Therapists," ©2001 American Massage Therapy Association.

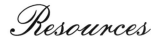

Sources of Information About Third-party Reimbursement

- Callahan, Margery M. and David W. Luther. *The Medical Massage Office Manual*. Parker, CO: CompMed Billing, 1998.
- Dolan, David. *Insurance Reimbursement & Specialty Physician Referrals: A Complete Reference for Massage and Physical Therapists*. Santa Barbara, CA: American Health Press, 1998.
- Fleetwood, Mary Anne. "A Program to Get Those Elusive Insurance Reimbursement Dollars." *Massage Therapy Journal,* Spring/Summer 1997.
- Rosche, Christine. *The Insurance Reimbursement Manual for America's Bodyworkers, Bodytherapists and Massage Professionals*, Fifth Edition. Palo Alto, CA: Bodytherapy Business Institute, 1998.
- Thompson, Diana L. *Hands Heal: Communication, Documentation, and Insurance Billing for Manual Therapists*. Lippincott Williams & Wilkins, 2001.

Time Management

Massage therapy enhances people's health and well-being. But for a massage therapist, it can be hard on the body. So if you want to be truly successful, you must set aside time to take care of yourself, including your body, mind, and spirit.

Chapter 6 talks about the importance of taking care of yourself. Consider the time for self-care as a primary business commitment, and place a high priority on it when it comes to scheduling your day's activities. Managing your personal and family lives is an important part of recognizing your wholeness. Remember that the word health comes from the Old English word *hal*, meaning "whole." If we want to be healthy, we must take care of our whole selves. If you are well rested and clearheaded, you will provide better massages and be more attuned to your clients' wants and needs. Likewise, you will be better able to handle work-related stress if you have solid support from your family, friends, and religious or spiritual community.

Each of us has the same amount of time—twenty-four hours in every day. Whether we are satisfied with our work depends in part on how we spend those twenty-four hours. Time management involves making conscious choices about time. For example, you can allow extra time between appointments for catching up with late arrivals. Or, you can let everyone know you have a policy that when someone's late arrival interferes with another appointment, you have to shorten the late person's session.

One basic tool of time management is the to-do list. It helps you decide what tasks you need to do and which of those tasks is most important. Allowing, of course, for surprises, you focus on the most important task first. An example of a way to manage your time using a to-do list follows:

1. *Weekly activities list*—Each week, list the activities you would like to accomplish during that week. Include the tasks you must accomplish, as well as those that you simply hope to complete.
2. *ABC ranking*—Next to each item that you believe is essential to your career or personal life, write an A. Mark items that are important but not essential with a B and remaining items with a C.
3. *Scheduling*—Block out time in your schedule for the A-level items on your list. Schedule this time as early in the week as possible, in case something unexpected forces you to reschedule them.
4. *A-level tasks*—Get started on the A-level items. Try not to think about the other tasks on your list. If something comes up, see if you can work it into your list; decide whether it is more important than your current A-level project.
5. *B- and C-level activities*—When you cannot do an A-level activity, do something you marked B; when you cannot do a B-level activity, do something you marked C.
6. *Reevaluation*—If something remains on your to-do list for longer than four weeks, reevaluate it. Is it something you really need to do? Can someone else do it? Should you just take it off the list altogether?

When you make a to-do list and rank activities, keep all your goals in mind. For example, if you want to enjoy your work and your life, you have to allow time for rest. If you do not, you may have to list a nap as an A-level activity. Likewise, you cannot make writing SOAP notes a C-level activity simply because you do not enjoy doing it; you have to fulfill your obligations to do the paperwork related to your work. However, you can break up some tasks that seem overwhelming. For example, if you run your own practice, you might not want to make writing a policy manual an A-level activity, but writing a particular section of it might be ranked as A-level. And remember, on some days the most important thing you do will be listening to someone or taking a walk and coming up with a great idea.

Another basic tool of time management is the calendar or appointment book. Entering your activities onto a calendar can help you remember what you need to do and avoid or resolve conflicts. It will also help you put your to-do list into action.

Suppose, for example, you are working from the previous to-do list. You enter the A-level activities on your calendar, then add the B-level activities. You observe that if you attend the Toastmasters meeting (a B-level activity), you will be hard-pressed to arrive for your first massage appointment (an A-level activity) in a relaxed, focused frame of mind. So you decide to skip the meeting this time and instead use the time for yoga, something you consider essential to your physical and spiritual health.

See the "Sample Daily 'To Do' List" (figure 3.27, page 166) for a sample of a well-planned and well-balanced massage therapist's day. Keep in mind that your priorities may shift; it may be necessary to reassign rankings when circumstances change.

Figure 3.27: Sample Daily "To Do" List

To Do
○
A— 30 minutes for yoga at 7:30 a.m.
A— 60-minute massage for Carole at 9:30 a.m.
A— 30-minute massage for Tom at 12:15 p.m.
B— Write outline for next week's speech
C— Straighten supply shelves
Etc.

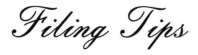

Filing Tips

Managing Paper
- File materials immediately.
- Files should be in use or put away.
- Put the most current materials in the front of the file.
- Label the file folder.
- Separate active files from archive files.
- Do not overstuff folders—create subfiles.
- Color-code files.
- Ease filing by reducing oversized documents to letter size.
- When a project is finished or a client is inactive, remove extraneous material from the file and archive it.

Organizing Computer Information
- Use the same names for directories, folders, and files that you label your paper documentation storage.
- Back up your files regularly, and store them in a fireproof box or preferably off premises.
- Each day delete unnecessary automatic back-up files.
- Eliminate inactive files on a monthly basis.

Source: Cherie Sohnen-Moe. "Taking Care of Business: Cleaning Up Your Office." *Massage Therapy Journal*, Spring 2000, pages 70, 72, 74, 78.

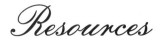

Sources and Ideas for Time Management Tools

- Go to your office supply store for a variety of calendars and scheduling tools
- Bly, Robert W. *101 Ways to Make Every Second Count: Time Management Tips and Techniques for More Success and Less Stress.* Career Press, Inc., 1999.
- Covey, Steven R., A. Roger Merrill, Rebecca R. Merrill. *First Things First Every Day Because Where You're Going Is More Important Than How Fast You're Going.* New York: Fireside, 1997.
- Franklin Covey Planner™: 1-800-655-1492; www.franklincovey.com

Employee Management

If you hire employees or enter into contracts for others to provide your practice with services, managing your practice will include managing the work of those people. This process begins with selection of qualified people. In addition, you must ensure that their work meets the standards you have established for your practice. For information about hiring employees, see "Hiring Employees" section in chapter 2 (page 74).

Once you have hired employees, it is your responsibility to clearly communicate their duties and your policies. You must be able to identify problem situations early to assist employees in correcting them. You must also have a plan in case an employee does not perform as expected and fails to improve.

Pay and Benefits

Your responsibilities to the employee also include compensating the employee through a combination of pay and benefits. The wage (hourly rate) or salary (weekly or monthly rate) you pay an employee is something the two of you agree on at the time you hire the employee. In addition, as shown in "Employee Pay and Benefits" (figure 3.28, page 168), employers provide benefits (some of which are required by law). When you decide what to pay an employee, keep in mind that as much as another ten to thirty percent of the employee's salary could go to expenses related to benefits.

Withholding Taxes

Federal and state income tax laws also impose requirements for employers to withhold taxes. Your practice is considered an employer if you hire anyone or if you incorporate. (If you incorporate and draw a salary, you are an employee of your practice.) If you are an employer, you must get an Employer Identification Number (EIN) from the IRS.

Whenever you hire employees, they should complete a W-4 form to specify their withholding allowances. Each quarter, you need to send the withholding amount to the IRS and/or state tax agency with the required form. In the case of federal income tax, you submit the check for income taxes, FICA (Social Security), and

---

Figure 3.28: Employee Pay and Benefits

Required by Law	*Optional Benefits*
Basic wage or salary or commission	Vacation pay
Matching employee's share of Social Security taxes (FICA)	Sick pay
Overtime pay for work beyond forty hours per week	Disability coverage
Federal and state unemployment taxes	Health insurance
Workers' compensation insurance	Life insurance
	Retirement plans

Note: Check with your state's labor department to find out which benefits are required in your state.

Medicare taxes with Form 941. The amount of income tax you withhold will depend on the tax rate and the withholding allowances claimed by the employee. For Social Security and Medicare taxes, the employer withholds 7.65 percent from the employee's pay and also pays another 7.65 percent as the employer's share. Self-employed people, in contrast, pay the full 15.3 percent themselves.

Then, by January 31 of the following year, you must send each employee Form W-2. This form shows the employee's total earnings and the amount withheld for each kind of tax. State withholding schedules and forms vary, so check with your state's tax agency.

Educating yourself ahead of time is important protection from the penalties for failure to comply with tax laws and regulations.

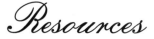

Resources

Guidelines for Withholding and Wage Reporting
- The Social Security Administration (1-800-772-6270 or www.ssa.gov) provides online information, an information kit, and a service center to answer questions about wage reporting.
- IRS Publication 15, *Circular E: Employer's Tax Guide*, details how to meet federal regulations.
- Your state's department of revenue has information about state withholding requirements.

Working Conditions

Employers must provide a safe and healthful workplace. Keeping the practice area clean and sanitary protects employees as well as clients. Employees should understand the importance of washing their hands, disinfecting equipment, and other basics of hygiene and sanitation. In addition, solvents and chemicals used in the practice must be stored properly, according to directions on the container.

A primary issue facing massage therapists is repetitive strain injuries, such as carpal tunnel syndrome. Chapter 6 contains information on how to prevent repetitive strain injuries. Employers should ensure that employees take such precautions. It is important for employees who spend hours at a computer each day to have ergonomically correct chairs and desks, and to regularly take breaks to avoid eye, wrist, and back strain.

Motivating Employees and Independent Contractors

A smart employer provides motivation, especially by observing employees' work and praising their accomplishments. When there is more than one person, "team play" creates a successful practice.

As an employer, you set the tone of your practice. Let your employees know how you like to operate so they can be part of the team. This involves various aspects of motivation. Motivation theories indicate that motivation involves several issues related to employee needs and expectations:

Employee Needs and Expectations	*Employer Responsibilities*
Employees expect fair compensation for their work, plus reasonably safe and pleasant working conditions.	Employers must provide fair pay and benefits and safe working conditions.
Employees do best if they understand what is expected of them.	Employers need to select people who are capable of learning the job, and they may need to provide some training as well.

(list continues on next page)

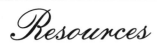

Guidelines for Supervising Employees

- Belker, Loren B. *The First-Time Manager, Fourth Edition.* New York: AMACOM Books, 1997.
- Broadwell, Martin M. *The New Supervisor: How to Thrive in Your First Year as a Manager, Fifth Edition.* Reading, MA: Perseus Books, 1998.
- Kilmer, Beverly. *Salon Ovations' Staffing Policies & Procedures.* Albany, NY: Milady Publishing, 1996.
- Sohnen-Moe, Cherie. "Practice Management, Part I." *Massage Therapy Journal*, Fall 1997.

Employees do best if they have some control over the resources they need to achieve their goals.

Employers need to provide clear directions and to check whether employees understand them.

Employers must be sure they understand what employees need, and provide access to those resources, such as supplies, petty cash, or authority to give refunds to unhappy clients.

Meeting these guidelines requires continuous two-way communication between you and your personnel. Block out time in your schedule to meet regularly with your employees, individually and as a group. Also schedule annual or more frequent performance appraisals. During the meetings and appraisals, be sure to listen as well as talk to your employees. Ask what they need in order to do their jobs better or enjoy their work more. This can be a rich source of valuable information to both of you. Use the process as a positive planning effort that is not punitive in any way.

Employee Policies

If you have employees, you can help them succeed by being clear about what you expect. You and they will need to know when they are expected to be at the office. They will also appreciate being able to refer to your practice's policy manual to see what benefits you are providing, including the schedule for performance appraisals.

Employee policies will include such topics as tipping and wages, work hours and days off, benefits, dress and hygiene requirements, reasons for dismissal, and competition from other employees. Your policy manual can be viewed as a legal document, so have your attorney review it before you distribute it. See the section "Policy Setting" (chapter 5, page 216) for more information about the types of employee policies you might consider for your business.

Non-compete Agreement

If your employees or contractors include other massage therapists, you may want policies with a non-compete clause or information that indicates who retains clients when an employee leaves his or her position. A non-compete clause may simply forbid employees from taking on any of your current clients. An alternative is a penalty finder's fee to compensate you for any clients you lose. (A non-compete clause forbidding a former employee or contractor from starting a similar business within a set number of miles may not stand up in court.)

Many massage therapists believe there is so much unmet demand for massage that building professional relationships is more important than worrying about this type of competition. In any event, the client and therapist have formed a therapeutic relationship, so be sure to allow for closure between them. Ultimately, clients will make the final decision to see the massage therapist with whom they feel most comfortable.

Who Owns Client Records?

Related to the topic of non-compete clauses is the larger issue of who owns client records. Clients have the right to seek care from the practitioner of their choice. The client completes an intake form on his or her first visit to a practitioner. In the United States, if the practitioner is an independent contractor who rents space and maintains client records independently, the practitioner owns the client record. If the practitioner is an employee, the business owns the client record.

As a former employee, you would not be entitled to take any client records with you if you were no longer employed by that business. If you signed a non-compete agreement, you could not ethically seek business from your former employer's clients. Clients are free, however, to choose the practitioners they prefer, and if one continued as your client, you would ask him or her to complete a new client intake form.

The Health Insurance Portability and Accountability Act (HIPAA) will also affect how you use client records in the United States. For more information, see "HIPAA" section on page 161.

The rules are different in Canada, where by law the information on the client intake form belongs to the client. Some provinces (Ontario, for instance) require massage practitioners to retain access to client records for 10 years. This means that massage practitioners must either retain the records themselves, or must sign an agreement with the employer that allows the practitioner to have continued access to client records in accordance with the province's requirements.

Client Scheduling

Records of how you plan to use your time take the form of schedules. Schedule your time and your appointments carefully, so that you will be ready for your clients when they arrive for an appointment. This is an important part of professionalism. If you will travel to appointments, allow plenty of time for traffic and to set up. Also, if you will see a series of clients at one location, be sure to allow about 30 minutes between appointments to change linens, get a drink of water, make notes about your previous client, and give your hands an ice bath.

Appointment Schedules

To stay organized and be ready for clients, you will need to keep records of appointments. Unless you have only a handful of clients, you will need a more formal system than a basic calendar. Purchase an appointment book and keep it near the telephone. Be sure to mark out the times you are not available. Whenever someone calls to set up, change, or cancel an appointment, record the appointment immediately.

If callers cannot see you at one of your available times, refer them to another massage therapist. As clients come in, let them know you will give them the same time slot for their next appointment if they prefer to schedule in advance. This way, you save appointment times that are convenient for them.

Typically, an appointment book has a week's worth of dates arranged in columns or blocks on each two-page spread. Make sure your appointment book has enough space to mark changes and still be readable. For each date, time intervals such as hours or half hours usually are marked. You write the client's name and phone number in the appropriate space or spaces so that the total length of the appointment is indicated. Colored pencils are best to use for marking an appointment book because they allow you to associate a color with a different activity or person using the massage room. Also, for a client's first visit, be sure to schedule additional time for the intake interview.

If you have an employee who records appointments, you will need to provide him or her with guidelines for allowing time between appointments. Instruct your employee to schedule at least thirty minutes for rest, cleanup, and preparation between clients.

Handling Phone Calls

Setting up appointments requires phone skills as well as an appointment book. Of course, you cannot sit by the phone all day yourself, so you need a plan for how to handle phone calls:

- You could use voice mail or an answering machine to record messages. This is the easiest arrangement, but consider how your clients will react to getting a recording.
- You could use an answering service. This costs a little more, but it ensures your clients will talk to a person and not a machine. A good answering service can handle calls in a professional manner. If you use one, provide appropriate information and training to assure that the service is very familiar with your business. Just as you do with other outside services, get referrals. Occasionally test the service by calling your office and letting the service answer. Do you like the way they handle your call before they know it is you calling?
- You could carry a pager and give your clients a pager number. This may be useful if you have clients with urgent needs. However, it has the disadvantage that clients will have to reach a device rather than a person.
- You could carry a mobile phone at all times, though you still will need a plan for what to do if your phone rings during an appointment. You should not interrupt the appointment to answer the phone. You would become distracted, and your client might feel put off.
- You could hire a receptionist to answer your phone during business hours. This enables you to establish your own guidelines for quality of client service, but it is also the most costly solution. It makes the most sense for a large practice or a situation in which you are sharing space and the receptionist with other professionals. If you are sharing the receptionist's services, you will have to agree on to whom the receptionist will report.

Shared Wisdom

"It's been my experience that, even when someone else is available to answer the phone at my practice, clients prefer to talk with me personally when they call to book an appointment. It might not be the most efficient way to schedule appointments, but I think my willingness to honor the client's preference to book with me personally helps strengthen our therapeutic relationship and promote ongoing business with those clients."

—*Ian Kamm, Sutherland-Chan School and Teaching Clinic, Toronto, Canada*

Answering the Call

Rachel McKinley, a massage therapist in Eau Claire, Wisconsin, got fed up with her answering machine. She would hear the phone ring during a massage session. But when she checked her messages afterward, nothing was there. Apparently her clients did not want to discuss their needs with a machine.

McKinley took matters into her own hands by setting up her own answering service. She started her business, called My Receptionist, to handle calls for massage therapists nationwide. The ten staff members take messages—for McKinley and her answering service clients—schedule appointments, and even call clients to remind them of upcoming appointments. In addition, they are trained to answer basic questions related to massage therapy and the fees charged.

The cost of the answering service is $29.95 each month, plus an additional 70 cents for each minute of calling time beyond the first ten minutes. The rates must be appealing. After just a year of operation, My Receptionist already was serving eighty massage therapy practices.

Source: Kelle Walsh. "May I Take a Message?" *Massage Magazine*, September/October 1998, page 184.

The skills required to manage all the administrative tasks of a well-run massage therapy practice cannot be undervalued. An administrative approach that functions smoothly, with a minimum of bottlenecks and last-minute crisis management, allows you to improve your profitability and to project a sense of competence and ease to your clients.

Chapter Summary

Learning to operate a business that serves its clients well and also yields a profit requires good skills in financial management, client records management, and administrative management.

Keys to good financial management include keeping accurate records that allow you to create financial statements that help you see the health of your business in terms of how much money you're receiving and how much you're expending. Good financial control systems can alert you to danger signs and allow you to take corrective action, such as cutting back on expenses or seeking more paying clients.

Gaining the advice of an accountant or tax specialist is especially important if you are self-employed. A specialist can help you determine how much you owe in quarterly estimated tax payments, and can help you identify allowable business tax deductions.

Equally important to financial management is your management of client records. Client records include: client intake form, informed consent statement, release of information approval, SOAP charts, client follow-up, and client visits and billing records. This information allows you to provide responsible health care to the client, and also gives you an opportunity to educate the client about what to expect in your massage sessions. Keeping accurate client records also allows you to see trends in your growth or decline of client visits so that you can modify your marketing tactics to fit your business needs.

Administrative management skills are necessary in order to maintain the financial and client records required for your business. If you choose to accept third-party reimbursement clients whose insurance benefits pay for all or part of their visits, you will need to set up an administrative system that helps you operate a referral system with other healthcare providers. You will also need to submit claim forms to insurance companies and track receipt of third-party reimbursement payments.

Other administrative tasks necessary to running your business include good time management, efficient filing systems, and responsible employee management. Your responsibility to employees includes paying certain payroll taxes, as well as complying with other state and national employment laws.

Once your management systems are in place and your method of recordkeeping is organized, you may find that the paperwork requirements of running your business provide a different type of satisfaction to you than your client care does.

Review Questions

1. What basic financial business records and statements are relevant to the management of a massage therapy practice?

2. What client records are necessary to your massage practice?

3. What communications strategies are appropriate for networking effectively and building relationships with other healthcare professionals in the care of shared clients?

4. What administrative management practices are necessary to the operation of massage therapy business?

5. What legal considerations affect your business if you have employees?

6. Name three advantages to hiring a professional accountant to assist you with financial and tax management.

4

CREATING *a* SENSE *of* PLACE

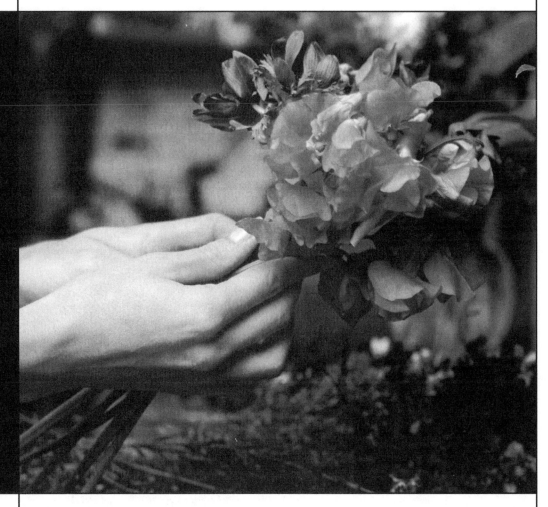

YOUR TOUCH OF THE CLIENT BEGINS LONG BEFORE YOU APPLY YOUR HANDS. UNDERSTAND THE MESSAGES YOU SEND AND HOW THEY AFFECT YOUR RELATIONSHIP WITH CLIENTS.

Chapter Objectives

1. Identify the physical components of a session space.

2. Describe the factors that make a session space appropriate to the client.

3. Make decisions related to the therapeutic environment, considering client preferences.

4. Identify ways to compensate for session space that is not ideal.

The physical environment in which you practice communicates messages to your clients on multiple levels. In this chapter we will look at the components that will make up your physical practice space, and how those components create the image you will want them to.

The Clients' Perspective

When you begin the process of choosing physical space for your future practice, look at space from your potential clients' point of view and consider how the decisions you make will affect their perception of your practice. At every point of client contact, consider all the senses—what the client will see, hear, smell, and touch. Consider, too, the physical and mental ease with which the client will encounter your business—will it seem professional? welcoming? intimidating? safe? awkward? competent?

As a potential client drives or walks by your business:
Will your signage be visible from the street?
What image will your signage convey—clinical, luxurious, modern, holistic?
Will the entrance into the building be welcoming? into your office space
    (if not the same as the building's entry)?
Will neighborhood smells be apparent, such as a chocolate factory or a
    pig farm?
Will it be on a busy thoroughfare or on a quiet, tree-lined lane?
Will it be easy to get to with public transportation?
Will neighboring businesses attract the same type of client you want to attract?

As a client arrives at your office:
Will your business be easy to find?
Will parking be available?
Will entry to your building and to your office be free of obstruction?
Will entry to your building and to your office space be well-lighted?
Once in the lobby of the building, will a directory or sign easily identify
    which office is yours?

As a client enters and waits in your reception area:
Will the area be well-lighted?
Will it be clean?
Will the entry to your office be accessible by a person in a wheelchair?
Will there be a convenient area to leave outerwear, boots, and umbrellas?
Will any fragrances be apparent? (This could be perceived as positive by
    some clients and as a drawback by others.)
What sounds will be heard in the reception area? music? voices from session
    rooms?
When the phone rings, will a receptionist or an answering machine answer?
If an answering machine, will the caller's voice be heard?
If the client needs to fill out paperwork, will pens and writing surfaces be
    handy?

If the client has a question, will the office layout make it easy for him or her to ask it privately before the session begins?

Will ventilation provide healthy air quality and movement?

What will the client see on your office walls? art? professional association member certificate? credentials? code of conduct? standards of practice? credos? building safety instructions?

Will the waiting area furniture be comfortable?

What reading materials will be available to clients as they wait?

Will water or other beverages be available?

If you will sell products, will they be displayed attractively where clients can access them?

Will rest room locations be marked clearly?

As a client enters your session space:

Will music be playing?

Will the temperature in the room be comfortable for the client?

Will a screen be available for client privacy?

Will the massage table already be made up attractively with clean linens?

Will lighting be indirect but sufficient for the client to undress and dress?

Will there be hooks on the walls and surface areas for the client to put his or her clothes and accessories?

Will a chair be available for the client's comfort and safety in removing shoes, etc.?

Will tissues and a wastebasket be handy for the client's convenience?

If there's a window in the room, will it offer privacy from outside view?

Will the décor of the space be restful or otherwise appropriate?

Will voices or other noises from outside the practice space be heard?

As a client leaves your session space:

Will water be available if your client wants it?

Will lighting be sufficient to help the client move around safely?

Will a basin of warm water and washcloth and towel be available?

Will a mirror be available?

Will all obstructions be removed for the client's safe exit from the space?

As a client leaves your office or building:

Will there be a convenient area in which the client can make payment for the massage and to book the next appointment?

Will a monthly calendar be available to make it easy for the client to re-book?

Will your business cards be visible for the client's convenience in passing your name along to a friend?

If other clients are waiting in the lobby, will there be adequate seating for everyone to be comfortable?

See "Complying with the Americans with Disabilities Act" (figure 4.1, page 180) for more details on physical space requirements.

If your answer to any of these questions indicates that the location is not appropriate, as it currently exists, for a good massage therapy practice, can you identify strategies that would neutralize your concern? The section "Office Space Variations," on page 186, discusses possible approaches for adapting less than ideal office space to your needs.

Your Perspective as a Business Owner

In the first part of this chapter, you considered potential office space from your clients' perspective. It is equally important to ask questions from the perspective of a business owner. Your clients' perspective is, naturally, a major factor in the decisions you make as a business owner, but there are many other factors to consider also.

Choosing Your Location

This section pertains to situations in which you are planning to rent or lease your own space for your massage business. Other options include: using space at another place of business, such as chiropractic or physical therapy office; outcall massage at clients' homes; at an employer's location; shared space with an existing massage therapy practice. For information on space considerations when you do not own or lease your own space, see the section "Office Space Variations" on page 186.

Start your search for office space by identifying the general area in which you want to practice. Once you have selected an area, you will need to determine whether it is suitable for your practice. Consider business and regulatory issues as well as your own comfort level and general appeal of the neighborhood. You will spend many hours at your place of business, and your satisfaction with your space will help you provide an optimum environment for your clients.

Contact the area's economic development office and ask for information about starting a business there. Ask such questions as:
- What are the zoning regulations? (Have an expert, such as a zoning officer or real estate attorney, determine whether your practice would be compatible with the zoning ordinances. Even a minor zoning change can take weeks or months. Also, zoning ordinances change, so even if a similar practice is in the same space or nearby, it does not mean you can set up a new practice there.)
- What will you need in the way of business licenses and permits?
- Are there tax considerations you need to be aware of?
- Is census or population demographic information available that would help you identify client demand?
- How many other massage practitioners have businesses that serve this area's population? (For a more detailed discussion of calculating supply and demand, see "Estimating Supply and Demand" [chapter 2, page 55].)
- Is there a local business association that charges dues or a government requirement for additional taxes to operate in this area?
- Are businesses in this area expected to be open (or closed) during certain hours?
- Is the location near services you need or would enjoy? For example, is there somewhere to do your laundry if your washer breaks down? Is there somewhere pleasant you can go for a juice or coffee break?
- Will you feel safe working in this neighborhood?
- Will your commute to and from home be convenient?

Choosing Your Office Space

To choose a specific office building within that area, you can either visit locations that might work for you and jot down the names of leasing agents on signs advertising vacancies, or you could find a real estate agent first and let him or her identify available locations. Ask your mentor, colleagues, and other small-business owners to recommend a helpful agent (preferably one who knows what massage therapy is about). Before you use that person's services, ask about his or her fee.

Also consider using the services of an attorney. Commercial leases may lack the consumer protection of a residential lease. Find an attorney who is familiar with the practice of leasing space for a business. This person can review your lease agreement and educate you about your options, such as whether utilities should be included in the rent, whether the lease will allow cost increases, the length of time of the lease, and other expenses associated with the lease. The savings and peace of mind you achieve with a well-drafted lease agreement may more than make up for the attorney's fee.

When you identify a space that interests you, get to know it. Visit the area two or three times during the hours you plan to operate your practice. Each time, stay thirty or forty minutes and observe the environment (light, air, noise, drafts, smells, traffic).

As you narrow your selection to a particular office site, ask such questions as:
- Are nonsmoking ordinances in effect for all or part of the building?
- Are the terms of the lease acceptable and in line with standard practice for the area? For example, the landlord should be able to tell you not only the length of the lease but how much you will have to spend for rent (per square foot), utilities, and parking or other fees, including breaking the lease (opting out of the space before the lease expires).
- Will the landlord allow or build out bathroom facilities, a wash basin with hot and cold running water, and hookups for your washer and dryer?
- What will it cost to maintain the space? Include carpet cleaning, garbage pickup, and snow removal, if these apply.
- Is construction of other space within the building planned that would be disruptive to your sessions?
- What provisions has the landlord made for safety and security?

You must also consider the interior space of your prospective office, including its amenities. As you review the space, evaluate space for giving massages and handling business activities, and evaluate the reception area. Ask questions such as the following:
- Are you able to control the temperature adequately? (Remember, massage clients will have greater needs for warmth than, say, customers of a store.)
- What security features and services does the building owner provide? For security issues that could affect your business, see "Security and Safety Considerations" (figure 4.2, page 181).
- Are there adequate electrical outlets and wiring for your needs? Will you be able to operate your computer, clothes dryer, or any other electrical equipment?
- Is there a sink or adequate plumbing to install one?
- Is there a bathroom available for you and your clients?

- Is the space compatible with the Americans with Disabilities Act? (See figure 4.1, below.)
- Will the landlord make changes you need (e.g., building out plumbing)? Who will pay for them? (Often costs are shared between landlord and tenant.)
- If there were ever a loss to report, what would the landlord's insurance cover?
- Does the office space meet accessibility standards?

Whatever you do, wait to sign a lease until you learn these important facts. Review all the facts you have gathered with your attorney or with a trusted mentor before making a final decision.

Safety and Security Precautions

Especially for a home office, but also applicable to any office environment, you must be prepared for unpredictable situations and emergencies. Before you invite any clients to your office, complete the checklist shown in "Security and Safety Considerations" (figure 4.2, page 181). This is also a good checklist to review periodically.

Figure 4.1 Complying with the Americans with Disabilities Act

In 1990, Congress passed the Americans with Disabilities Act (ADA), which requires businesses serving the public to make their facilities accessible to people with disabilities. (In addition, if you hire employees, the workplace must be accessible to them.) Here are some tips for making your space accessible to your clients:

- Get standards from the U.S. Department of Justice (1-800-514-0301 or www.usdoj.gov)

- Remember that disability does not just mean "in a wheelchair." Other disabilities include sight or hearing impairment, arthritis, and heart conditions.

- Think about the client types you are targeting. Will certain physical limitations be more likely among this group? Are you prepared to accommodate clients with such conditions?

- Plan how a person with a physical disability will enter your office, pass through doorways, and move on and off the massage table. Are there steps? Are doorknobs easy to turn? (Use levers rather than knobs if you can.)

- Make sure it is easy to move around the space. Are chairs easy to get in and out of? Are floors easy to walk on? Avoid slippery, shiny surfaces (causing glare), or those covered with obstacles, such as electrical cords or small rugs.

Figure 4.2

SECURITY AND SAFETY CONSIDERATIONS

Physical Safety Features

❏ I have checked the sidewalk and entrance to my office for obstacles and toe catches.

❏ I assure that all ice and snow is cleared prior to my first appointment.

❏ I have seen and approved the building maintenance and cleaning plan (if managed by an independent building supervisor).

❏ I keep stairways and hallways free of clutter.

❏ I have checked the stability of railings.

❏ I keep throw rugs to a miniumum, and make sure the ones I have do not present safety risks. (I do not use throw rugs if I practice massage on elderly or clients with physical disabilities.)

❏ My massage table is stable and in good repair.

❏ I maintain a log book of equipment inspections.

Medical Preparedness

❏ I have learned to administer first aid, including CPR.

❏ I have a first-aid kit easily available in my office.

❏ I remind clients to dispose of candy or gum before they get on the massage table.

❏ I practice universal precautions as standard procedure in my office.

Personal Security

❏ I have an emergency buzzer or other system installed in case I need to call for help.

❏ I screen my clients and verify that they are clear about the nature of the service I provide. (Many experienced massage therapists recommend accepting new clients only when referred by someone else.)

❏ I have a plan for handling inappropriate comments or behavior by clients.

❏ I follow a procedure for letting someone know who I am scheduled to see and when.

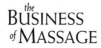

© 2002 American Massage Therapy Association, Evanston, IL. *The Business of Massage.* All Rights Reserved. #20026

Costs of Office Space

When you consider leasing a space, know all the costs involved. In the "Career and Practice Planning Worksheet" (chapter 2, figure 2.24, page 102), see the financial section for details about costs you should anticipate in starting and operating your practice. The cost of office space could be one of your largest expenses. Before you sign a lease, decide whether you can afford it by identifying the initial and monthly expenses of space, as follows:

One-time Initial Costs
Cost to prepare space (painting, decorating, bringing into
compliance with ADA, upgrading plumbing or electricity): $_____
Fees for real estate agent: $_____
Fees for attorney: $_____

Total initial cost to find and prepare leased space: $_____

Monthly Costs
Monthly rent: $_____
Monthly utilities not included in rent: $_____
Monthly taxes or fees for using space: $_____
Shared monthly or seasonal costs of maintaining common space
(such as snow removal or janitorial services): $_____

Monthly cost of space: $_____

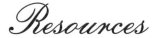

Ideas for Locating and Setting Up Office Space

- Martin Ashley, "Opening a Massage Office: A Step-by-Step Plan," *Massage Magazine* (March/April 1999).
- Cherie Sohnen-Moe, "Choosing and Designing Your Office Space," *Massage Therapy Journal* (Winter 1994).
- Greg Boddy, "Look Before You Lease," *Newsletter of the Ontario Massage Therapist Association* (August/September 1996).
- Robb Sykes, "Choosing a Location for Your Practice, Part I," *Newsletter of the Ontario Massage Therapist Association* (June/July 1996).
- Robb Sykes, "Choosing a Location for Your Practice, Part II-Narrowing Your Search," *Newsletter of the Ontario Massage Therapist Association* (August/September 1996).
- Cherie Sohnen-Moe, "Zoning: Your Rights and Responsibilities," *Massage Therapy Journal* (Winter 1996).

Equipping Your Space

When we consider physical components, we mean more than just the building your business is housed in and the equipment and furniture that fill your office and session space. We are talking about all the tangible attributes that make up your business. As your client enters your space, it conveys to him or her certain expectations of the quality of massage to follow.

Your decisions about the image of your practice will depend largely on the type of client you are serving. If your practice specializes in medical or sports massage, its décor will differ from a practice whose clients are mostly interested in relaxation and stress reduction. A clinical atmosphere might be conveyed through such effects as white walls and stainless steel fixtures, whereas pastels and crystals convey a more holistic atmosphere. As your clients walk through your doors, you want them to feel an immediate sense of confidence that your practice suits their needs and expectations.

Furniture and Equipment

Massage therapists need two kinds of furniture and equipment for the practice: 1) items for providing massage, and 2) items for office work. "Equipping Your Massage Therapy Practice (figure 4.3, page 184) identifies furniture, equipment, and supplies that a typical practice needs.

Fortunately, you do not have to spend a fortune on office equipment. You could find a lovely desk at a garage sale or flea market, and used-equipment suppliers may have just the items you need. However, do consider your comfort and that of anyone else who will be using the equipment. Take into account ergonomic principles and how they can help you in a profession that is physically demanding already. Realize that you do not have to outfit the ideal office from day one. Make a list of the things that are essential to your practice and which ones will enhance it further, and plan your budget accordingly.

Supplies

Besides the big items of furniture and equipment, you also will have to stock the necessary supplies. "Equipping Your Massage Therapy Practice (figure 4.3, page 184) details many of the supplies needed by a typical massage therapy practice. If you will practice from an office, probably you will need most of these. If you will provide on-site massages, you must provide more than one or two items to be recognized as an independent contractor.

Over the course of several years, you will buy many office supplies, so it is worthwhile to identify one or more reliable sources of items you prefer to use. The office supply business is very competitive, and not all retailers are the same. Spend a few minutes calling stores listed in the business directory pages and ask each about discounts. Request a catalog. You may find that many of the largest chains have the most limited variety of items, and a smaller retailer that specializes in service may offer a much wider selection at about the same price. Buying in bulk can save you money in the long run, but be sure you have the space to store the supplies and that nothing will expire before you use it.

Shared Wisdom

"Keep your targeted client type in mind as you make decisions about your office design and image. A medical doctor once told me, 'I'm afraid that when I send a patient to an unknown massage therapist for a shoulder injury, they will have incense burning, music of whale sounds playing, and then stick a candle in the patient's ear and light it. I want to know that the therapist's office looks professional."

—*Bob Haase,*
Bodymechanics School of
Myotherapy & Massage,
Olympia, Washington

Figure 4.3

EQUIPPING YOUR MASSAGE THERAPY PRACTICE

For Office Use

FURNITURE/EQUIPMENT

- ❏ Desk
- ❏ Desk chair
- ❏ File cabinets
- ❏ Bookshelves
- ❏ Lamps
- ❏ Enclosed cabinet for linens and towels
- ❏ Storage cabinet for supplies
- ❏ Phones with automated answering system
- ❏ Waiting room furniture (chairs, tables, lamps, coat rack)
- ❏ Sink with hot and cold water
- ❏ Accessible toilet
- ❏ Soap dispenser
- ❏ Smoke detectors
- ❏ Fire extinguisher
- ❏ Carbon monoxide detector
- ❏ Computer and printer (optional)
- ❏ Copier (optional)
- ❏ Fax (optional)
- ❏ Display cases (optional)
- ❏ Step stool (optional)
- ❏ Small refrigerator (optional)
- ❏ Water cooler (optional)
- ❏ Electric hand dryer (optional)

Note: Refer to local zoning ordinances for additional needs

SUPPLIES

- ❏ Charts, forms, file folders
- ❏ Appointment book
- ❏ General ledger book
- ❏ Receipt books
- ❏ Message pads
- ❏ Follow-up folder
- ❏ Calculator
- ❏ Pens and pencils
- ❏ Paper (computer paper, copier paper)
- ❏ Stapler, staples, and staple remover
- ❏ Tape and tape dispenser
- ❏ Paper clips
- ❏ Ceramic or disposable cups
- ❏ Tea bags
- ❏ Ink, toner for printer, fax, copier (if you have this equipment)
- ❏ Software for computer (if you have computer)
- ❏ Diskettes for backing up computer files (if you have computer)
- ❏ Paper towels, toilet paper, antibacterial soap
- ❏ Cleaning supplies – window/mirror cleaner, cleanser for sink
- ❏ Disinfectant or fungicide for cleaning floors and any bath-area surfaces
- ❏ Oil-removing detergent (if you do not use a laundry service)
- ❏ First-aid kit

For Massage Therapy Use

EQUIPMENT

- ❏ Massage tables
- ❏ Linens, bolsters, pillows
- ❏ Massage chair (if you offer seated massage)
- ❏ Linen bin with lid
- ❏ Washer and dryer (if you do not use a laundry service)
- ❏ Stereo/CD player
- ❏ Cabinet for lotions and oils (optional)
- ❏ Space heater for session room (optional)

SUPPLIES

- ❏ Cassettes or CDs
- ❏ Lubricants and essential oils
- ❏ Clothing hooks and hangers
- ❏ Heated blankets and mattress pads (optional)
- ❏ Waist pack that holds massage oils or lotions (optional)
- ❏ Candles (optional)

the
BUSINESS
of MASSAGE

© 2002 American Massage Therapy Association, Evanston, IL. *The Business of Massage.* All Rights Reserved. #20026

Style and Layout of Furnishings

Another important aspect of setting up your space is to decorate for aesthetics and to convey the desired image of your practice. There is no one design approach that is right for every massage business. Some practitioners prefer clean and crisp lines and a modern silhouette to their reception area and session rooms. They might choose chrome and glass for the image they want to project. Others might gravitate toward a softer décor, in which they use wood furnishings and quilted coverlets. The only requirements for interior space are that it be safe and clean. As Nina McIntosh writes in *The Educated Heart*, "We want a balance between a room that smells antiseptic and a room that looks like germs may be lurking in every corner."

Aesthetic image of space is influenced by your choices of colors, textures, shapes, sounds, lighting, room layout, and art. Check each of the following features that are important to you, and indicate at least one way your décor can contribute to providing the image you want:

    Professionalism—provided with: _____
    Beauty—provided with: _____
    Relaxation—provided with: _____
    Health—provided with: _____
    Spirituality—provided with: _____
    Cleanliness—provided with: _____
    Safety—provided with: _____
    Other: _____—provided with: _____

One design philosophy that some massage practitioners have used in creating a therapeutic environment for themselves and their clients is feng shui. This Chinese ancient art is said to correct energy imbalances in the arrangement of one's space and the objects in it. See "Feng Shui and Clutter" for recommendations about how this design approach can help remedy a cluttered office space.

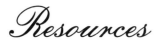

Where to Find Equipment and Supply Sources

- massage schools
- exhibitors at massage therapy conventions and meetings
- ads in professional magazines (such as *Massage Therapy Journal* and *Massage Magazine*)
- professional association chapters' newsletters
- Martin Ashley, *Massage: A Career at Your Fingertips, Third Edition* (Carmel, NY: Enterprise Publishing, 1999)—extensive appendix of equipment and supplies

Feng Shui and Clutter

One of feng shui's principle tenets is that clutter detracts from harmony. In *Clear Your Clutter with Feng Shui*, author Karen Kingston says there are four categories of clutter:

1. Things you do not use or love.

   Things that are loved or used and appreciated have strong vibrant and joyous energy around them. Things that are neglected, forgotten, unwanted, unloved, or unused will cause the energy to slow and stagnate. You are connected to everything around you by fine strands of energy. When you surround yourself with things you love, your environment supports you.

2. Things that are untidy.

   When things have a place and they are put there repeatedly, you know in your mind's eye their precise location. Lives work better when you know where things are. Energy strands get jumbled when your things are in a jumble, like tangled spaghetti.

3. Too much stuff in too little space.

   This is common when a business grows but the office doesn't. After filling up all its spaces, your office begins to feel as if it cannot breathe. Cabinets are full and passeageways are narrow. Doors cannot open. It's time to find new space or shift some of the stuff out.

4. Unfinished business.

   Things left unfinished clutter the psyche. Things not dealt with reflect issues not dealt with and drain your energy. Broken equipment, burned out light bulbs, outdated reading materials, all not only drain your energy but metaphorically remind you of unfinished and broken things inside. Best to fix them and let there be light!

Displaying Your Credentials

Some of the things you display may be required by law or ordinance. For example, if you are required to obtain a license, probably you will have to display it. Health laws or ordinances might specify signs or notices you must post in the restrooms. Displaying your license and other professional credentials such as your National Certification and professional association membership certificate are a simple but effective way to add to your professional image. Put professional credentials and the Code of Ethics in attractive frames and display them proudly. See the "Professional Credentials" section of chapter 2 (page 41), for more information about credentials and their proper use.

Office Space Variations

If money is no object, you will not have to worry about designing office space that fits your needs perfectly. However, most practitioners find that they must compensate for a gap between their ideal physical practice environment and reality. If you share space with another business, say a chiropractic office, a physical therapy clinic, or a beauty salon, you will work cooperatively with that business's personnel and policies. The same is true if you are employed by a spa, a fitness center, or a private practice, or if you practice on-site massage at a company's site.

The physical space in which you practice might meet many of your requirements but lack others. The room or rooms in which you have your sessions might be smaller than ideal or might not have suitable lighting. You might not have control over the room's thermostat. The room's décor might not be appropriate to a massage setting.

As you consider how to furnish your space in a way that meets your goals, take into account the people who will be using the space. If you are setting up a small office area for your use only, you can include anything that helps you work and leave out any distractions. Be considerate of others. If you will invite clients into this space, you must think about your clients' tastes and needs. A roomful of roses or incense may lift your spirits but may not be so appealing to someone with asthma or allergies. The same goes for scented oils. Whenever you can, provide choices in music so clients receive the nurturing they need.

One of the ways in which you naturally create your own identity is through your choice of linens, blankets, oils, bolsters, music, and other massage accessories. You might also consider taking your own space heater if you are concerned that the room's temperature will be too chilly for the client. To reinforce a professional atmosphere, your credentials should be displayed in a visible area. You might want to provide your own lamp that casts a soft light rather than use the overhead light already in the room. If privacy is a concern, you can devise a screen to cover a window.

If you work as an on-site massage therapist at another company's site, you have less influence over the massage environment, but there are still some things you can do. Take along a portable CD player and a few CDs. Take a single flower to place in a vase in the room where massages are provided. Arrive early to straighten up the clutter. Since you will not always know where you will be working, get in the habit of looking around the work area when you arrive. You may be able to contribute to the creation of a relaxing and aesthetically pleasing environment.

Go back to "The Clients' Perspective" section at the beginning of this chapter, and ask how your space stacks up against the considerations listed. Determine how you would compensate for the gaps between your ideal space and what is available. You must determine which limitations would seriously impact the way you prefer to work, versus those for which you can compensate in some way. If a location offers poor security or noise that would detract from a massage session, you might decide that those tradeoffs are too serious to accept. If, on the other hand, a potential office space has poor lighting, you might negotiate with the landlord to provide upgrades, or you could provide your own area lighting.

If you opt to start in space that clearly falls short of your ideal, all is not lost—your experience will help you clarify those things that are important to you, which you will choose when you can afford a different location.

Reevaluating Your Space

You will carefully analyze every aspect of your physical space requirements when you set up a business. It's important to review your space decisions on a regular basis to assure that they are still appropriate. When your lease expires is a good time to consider major changes, such as room layout, amenities that need to be added, or changes to the heating, air conditioning, and ventilation systems. These become negotiable items when you renew your lease.

Other design considerations you will want to review more frequently, such as every six months:

- Has your client focus changed in such a way that your décor no longer reflects their preferences and expectations?
- Are your framed credentials up-to-date?
- Is there a problem with traffic flow pattern that can be remedied without tearing down walls?
- Can you rearrange furniture in your reception area to make it more welcoming to clients?
- Do you need to revise your magazine subscriptions or brochures for client interest and education?

Consider asking your mentor or a regular client if he or she would be willing to give you feedback on what things work and don't work as far as your physical environment. If you have a client who has a specialty in space planning, who is accustomed to being compensated for this type of consultation, maybe you could barter for an exchange of services.

The key to having a physical environment that attracts clients is understanding your clients' needs and viewing your environment from their perspective. Taking the time to review those needs on a regular basis will pay off in client loyalty and in your own renewed commitment to operating a vital and healthy practice.

Chapter Summary

Whether you will be designing your own workspace or will be sharing space at an existing workplace, your choices about your physical surroundings will affect the success of your practice. When making decisions about office space, it is important to consider your clients' perspective as well as your own perspective as a business owner. Factors that will influence your selection of space include location, zoning ordinances, convenience, appearance, amenities, design, and cost.

Unless you have an unlimited budget, you will probably have to compromise on some of the features of your office space that fall short of your ideal. There are many ways in which you can compensate for limitations in your practice space, while still accommodating the personnel and policies of the office in which you work. Areas in which you can make a difference are in décor, comfort, and privacy for your clients. If you are an owner or renter of office space, it is important to be thorough in identifying all potential benefits, limitations and costs—initial as well as monthly—before signing a lease.

You will also have to select equipment and supplies for business and for massage use. When you complete your "Career and Practice Planning Worksheet" (introduced in chapter 2), you will decide how much and which equipment is essential to the start-up of your business, and which you can delay purchasing until later.

As long as you operate a profitable business, you will have the opportunity to continually improve and refine your physical space to your clients' and your own satisfaction.

Review Questions

1. Name three physical features of your office location or space that would influence a client positively or negatively.

2. What are three primary security and safety matters you must consider when establishing a massage therapy practice?

3. What kinds of decisions about your physical environment are related to the type of clients targeted by your business? (Targeted clients might be fitness, sports, medical, spa, wellness.)

4. What working environments could cause you to work in a less than ideal session space?

5. In what ways can you compensate for less than ideal space?

5

Creating *a* Therapeutic Relationship

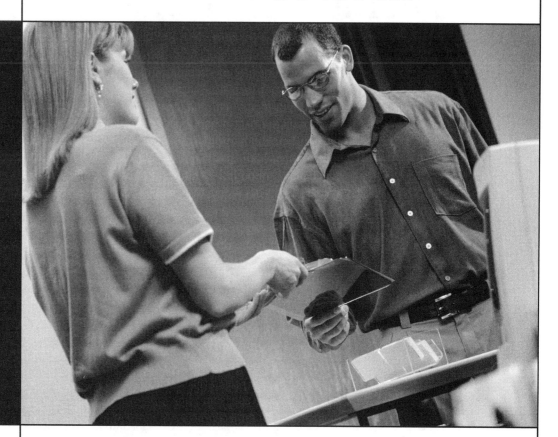

EXTEND THE SKILL OF YOUR HANDS EVEN FURTHER BY ACKNOWLEDGING AND NURTURING THE WHOLE PERSON WHO IS YOUR CLIENT.

Chapter Objectives

1. Describe the wellness model and distinguish between the wellness model and the medical model.

2. Identify the effect of language usage, vocabulary, style of speech, dress, posture, hygiene, and conduct on effective practitioner-client communication.

3. Describe the importance of instructing the client in self-care.

4. Identify practitioner behaviors that are consistent with confidentiality of client identification, personal disclosure, files, and treatment information.

5. Identify the roles, functions, and expectations of behavior of massage therapists in relation to common healthcare professional ethics.

6. Describe the process for establishing and maintaining professional boundaries and relationships with clients and peers in the workplace.

In a therapeutic environment, both you and your clients emerge healthier as a result of your session together than you were before the session. The effects of a therapeutic relationship between you and your clients are cumulative, and thus the benefits of your massages increase with each visit. This is good not only for the bodies, minds, and spirits of you and your clients, but good for your business as well. This chapter examines factors that contribute to or detract from a therapeutic relationship.

The Therapeutic Relationship

The essential quality of the interpersonal contact between client and practitioner is integral to determining the effectiveness of your massage work. As a professional, it is your responsibility to set the tone and the boundaries for ethical and compassionate care of your clients. If you are too hard-nosed and clinical, your clients will feel like units of profit. If you have fuzzy boundaries, your clients could think of themselves more as your friends than your clients. In either case, your clients would be unable to derive the full benefits of massage that are possible when a therapeutic relationship exists.

Common threads woven throughout the therapeutic relationship include adherence to ethical behaviors and codes of conduct, and sincerity and sensitivity in interpersonal communication skills. Elements intrinsic to a relationship that promotes wellness of the client and the practitioner include the following:

1. The whole presence of the therapist is critical to the therapeutic relationship. Presence includes the qualities of compassion, respect, non-judgment, unconditional acceptance, focus, mindfulness, and an attitude of friendly curiosity.
2. The practitioner's intuition and nurturing capabilities are essential, as are communication skills that may be learned. Guiding the therapeutic relationship requires both art and skill.
3. Practitioners do not fix or heal, but rather facilitate and empower the client's innate healing potential and ability to access the client's own wisdom.
4. Self-care is essential in renewing the practitioner's ability to work effectively.
5. Communication with others is reflective of the depth and clarity that the practitioner has of his or her own self. The personal growth work a practitioner does forms the basis for what he or she is able to offer clients.
6. The therapeutic relationship is non-sexual and is respectful of professional boundaries.
7. The quality of the therapeutic relationship between the practitioner and client is always ultimately the responsibility of the practitioner.
8. The therapeutic relationship functions within the legal boundaries of professional limitations and guidelines.

Adapted from *Kiné-Concept Institute Business Success Workbook*, by Barry Antoniow. Fredericton, New Brunswick, Canada: Kiné-Concept Institute Maritimes.

If you view these attributes within the context of the wellness model, described in the next section, it is easy to see how a good therapeutic relationship between a massage therapist and a client promotes the well-being of body, mind, and spirit.

The Wellness Model

Today, most massage therapists work within the wellness model. The wellness model views health as the sum total of a person's environment, which includes mind and spirit, as well as body. This is in contrast to the allopathic, or medical, model, which is based on the concept that health is achieved through the removal of disease. It would certainly be unfair to suggest that medical practitioners totally exclude the influences of mind and spirit on a person's health. By the same token, many massage therapy and bodywork practitioners, especially those who work in medical or sports settings, recognize when it is beneficial to focus particular attention on the physical body to promote relief of pain or discomfort.

Shared Wisdom
"By far the most useful business tool is understanding who your clients are—what is their model of the world, what do they believe in, how do they think, and what are their priorities in life? Point out to them—through your advertising, by how you dress, how you decorate your office—that you understand and respect them for who they are. In effect, meet them at their model of the world instead of expecting them to meet you at yours."

—*Craig McLaughlin, Mountain Heart School of Bodywork, Crested Butte, Colorado*

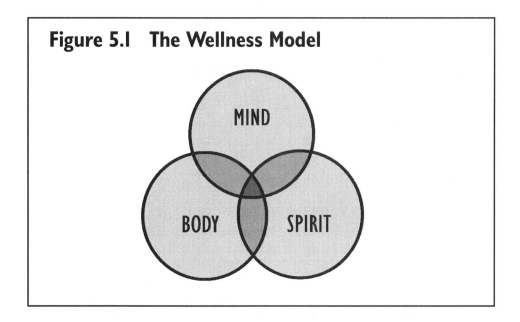

Figure 5.1 The Wellness Model

Several wellness models exist. The simplest model looks at a balance between mind, body, and spirit. Some models include the additional components of occupational, intellectual, and social. All models are based on the premise that it is necessary for an individual to achieve balance in his or her life in order to promote optimal health and well-being. All models capture the idea that all human factors and environments are interrelated. Rather than focusing on the part of the body that appears to be ailing, the wellness approach focuses first on prevention and on examining the balance of all related components. Is the person stressed? Is he or she getting enough sunshine? Is the person exercising regularly and drinking plenty of water? Does the person's daily routine provide a balance of work and leisure activities?

There is a wide range of difference in emphasis on one component or another, even within the wellness model, among massage therapists. The sports or medical massage therapist places a greater emphasis on body, while still acknowledging the intrinsic role that spirit and mind play in a person's health. The spirit and mind components are particularly valued and integrated into practice by the wellness massage therapist, who is also knowledgeable about and attentive to a client's physical body.

When you develop your referral networks with other healthcare practitioners (as described in chapters 3 and 7), it will be helpful for you to identify practitioners who have an appreciation for holistic approaches. They will be more open to including massage therapy in their recommendation to patients than will practitioners who strictly adhere to the medical model.

A Healing Modality

Consistent with the wellness model, the history of massage therapy and bodywork is rich in the tradition of healing. In *Persuasion and Healing*, author Jerome Frank, professor emeritus of psychiatry at Johns Hopkins University, identified four ingredients common to all healing modalities.

1. The client must feel confident of the practitioner's competence and desire to be of help.
2. The setting in which a session takes place must be designated by society as a place of healing or refuge, as distinguished from the client's regular environment.
3. The rationale of each therapeutic school of thought must explain the cause of distress, reveal desirable goals, and describe ways for attaining those goals. This strengthens the client's sense of empowerment and enables the client to make sense of what is happening within a therapeutic context.
4. The therapeutic procedure demands some effort or sacrifice on the part of the client. That is, there must be a transaction in which the client makes a sacrifice in return for the therapist's services, usually in terms of time and money, in order for the client to participate in his or her own healing.

Frank's work stated that when these four elements are present, favorable conditions are present for change. Items two and four above are mostly beyond the control of the massage therapist. But you have great influence over the degree to which items one and three affect your client. They are conveyed to the client through the practitioner's ability to communicate effectively.

Client Communications

Many of the elements of a therapeutic relationship described at the beginning of this chapter highlight the importance of effective communication skills. The fact that the therapeutic relationship is dependent on not only the practitioner's innate intuition, but also on skills that can be learned, encourages practitioners to hone their communication skills. This section identifies ways in which you, as a practitioner, can better understand how your verbal and non-verbal actions contribute to helping or harming your therapeutic relationship with a client.

Oral Communication Skills

Oral communication skills are essential for every massage therapist to develop. They are one of the most obvious tools to use in establishing themselves in relationship with clients. Most clients will not know the technical language of the massage therapy profession, and therefore general communication skills are required in order to put the client at ease.

When a client does not follow the practitioner's instructions, it could be due to the practitioner's inability to communicate clearly and skillfully. The success of oral communication depends on your ability to present information in a way that is understood accurately by the client, in facts as well as intent. The skills of conveying information, as well as listening, affect this success.

Vocabulary

Because your client probably will not know the technical vocabulary of massage, it is important that you learn to communicate using vocabulary that is clearly understood by the client. You have become accustomed during your training to communicate with peers who speak the language of massage, and it will take practice to convert this to language clients will understand.

This doesn't mean that you should be condescending in your explanations or that you should oversimplify them—after all, it is your role to help educate clients about the role and efficacy of massage. Mastery of appropriate vocabulary means knowing when and how to use professional jargon, and to translate it into everyday terms.

The goal of choosing appropriate vocabulary is to achieve desired results of the session, and to convey to the client that you are sincere in your desire to form a productive working client/therapist relationship with him or her.

Voice Clarity, Tone, and Volume

You know the adage: It's not what you say, it's how you say it. A highly organized, technically correct and meaningful sentence loses its impact when poorly articulated. Clients are often initially hesitant or sometimes intimidated in the presence of healthcare professionals. Your clarity of voice helps convey that you feel confident of the benefits you are about to impart, sincerely welcoming of the client, and professional in how you conduct your practice. Lack of voice clarity means that you mumble or slur your words, rather than clearly enunciate them. Lack of clarity suggests to the client that you are not confident of what you're saying. Clarity inspires trust.

Tone is a voice quality that can either reinforce or communicate exactly the opposite of the spoken words. A flat tone can convey indifference. A too-warm and soft tone can be misinterpreted as suggesting intimacy. A jovial tone might detract from a relaxation atmosphere, if that's what you're trying to create. It is important to be cognizant of tone not only when speaking but when listening. When a client's response is not clear or is surprising to you, be alert to the tone in which the client communicates or reacts to something you say. His or her tone might give you more clues to the actual meaning of the communication than words alone convey.

For instance, if a client says to you before starting a session, "I really need this today," her tone could indicate one of several meanings:

- She is in pain and needs special attention to a particular area. (Listen for emphasis on *really need*, and look for facial expression, such as wincing.)
- She is looking forward to a relaxation massage and enjoying this break from an otherwise hectic schedule. (Listen for lighthearted delivery or mock-seriousness.)
- She is stressed and is worried about taking the time for a massage because of all the other demands on her time. (Listen for sarcasm and an emphasis on the word *this*.)

If you are unclear about what the client means to say, it would be a good idea to simply ask for clarification. For instance, if you think the client has pain but hasn't said so, ask if he or she is having pain in any area.

Volume can be used to control distance between people. A soft whisper can make the listener move closer. It can also be used in a manipulative way, to control the listener's behavior by compelling him or her to lean toward you. Loud volume conveys aggression, or it can be an attention-getting device. You could send the wrong impression to your client if your voice were meek and faltering, or at the opposite extreme, if your voice were inappropriately loud.

Organization

The rambling practitioner confuses clients by jumping from one topic to the next, inserting last-minute ideas, and then failing to summarize or to ask the client to do so. Inability to progress from one step to the next and thereby reach a logical conclusion is usually due to:

- A lack of understanding of the topic or the steps in a procedure
- A too-thorough knowledge of the topic or procedure

The first instance—lack of understanding—would cause you to either grope for words or be at a loss for words since you're not sure what you want to say in the first place. The second instance—too-thorough knowledge—could cause you to give too much information to the client and to assume that the client has a need or interest to know more than is appropriate.

If you are communicating new information to a client, practice ahead of time how you will organize your thoughts and then your communication. It is a good idea to provide written instructions and diagrams whenever possible, to add to the clarity of your oral communication.

Sense of Humor

Injecting a sense of humor into the client/therapist relationship can help build rapport and trust quickly, but it also has its pitfalls. Whether you can use humor effectively with your client depends on your ability to accurately read your client's acceptance of humor. It also depends on the compatibility of your sense of humor and your client's. There is no one right or wrong way to use humor, because each instance is dependent upon the situation and the client and your own comfort with using humor.

Effective uses of humor might include:
- Reducing tension when it exists unnecessarily: "If I tickle you, you're allowed to laugh."
- Coaching for self-care: "I have a policy that limits me to one ski accident client a week, so be careful on the slopes this weekend."

Guard against destructive uses of humor, such as verbal fencing or sarcasm. It introduces animosity to the client/therapist relationship, and makes it difficult to enter into a healing atmosphere based on trust and comfort. If you find that you're tempted to use humor in order to avoid an uncomfortable confrontation, take a moment to think about a constructive way to communicate necessary information.

It is best to let the client set the tone of the communication, especially when you are in the early stages of establishing your relationship.

Adapted from *Kiné-Concept Institute Business Success Workbook*, by Barry Antoniow. Fredericton, New Brunswick, Canada: Kiné-Concept Institute Maritimes.

Listening Skills

Listening skills are as powerful, effective, and varied as are the skills of communicating orally. The two main goals of good listening skills are:
- To improve listening acuity so that the practitioner hears the client accurately
- To ascertain what a client has heard the practitioner communicate

Inability to listen effectively can be caused by several factors. The following factors are described to help you recognize when they apply to your own listening effectiveness, and also to acknowledge possible reasons why your client doesn't always hear the message you thought you delivered.

Mindset—The listener's past experiences or cultural background have created a particular mindset, or belief, about a topic. Such a belief might be, "It's not all right to have a stranger touch me." The client might not be consciously aware of this mindset and might communicate it in nonverbal ways, such as creating conflict or arriving late for appointments. A caution to be aware of here is that, unless you are a trained psychologist, do not attempt to interpret the client's responses in clinical terms. Simply being aware that what the client says and what the client means might be two different things is sufficient to your maintaining a healthy relationship with the client. Listening with a compassionate ear and striving for optimum well-being of both you and your client— not psychoanalyzing the client—is the goal.

Unrealistic expectations—If the client expects a certain result that is not likely to happen, the anticipation of that result could cloud the client's understanding of your words. For instance, if the client believed that the first session of a particular modality would totally remove a painful condition—and it didn't— the client might attribute that failure to your skills rather than realize that he or she was operating under unrealistic expectations. Further, if you did not determine that the client had these expectations, you would not even be aware that they should be addressed.

Sensory overload—The rate at which a listener can process incoming information depends on whether the listener is distracted by competing demands for his or her attention and by the rate at which the information is being conveyed. For instance, communicating effectively with a single parent who sandwiches in a massage for relaxation between childcare activities and a job might require extra sensitivity on your part to the client's distractions. When trying to cut through layers of distraction, your choice of vocabulary as well as your rate of speaking can help you convey information more effectively. Your awareness of a client's cultural background can also give you clues to whether the client is accustomed to such things as a fast or a slow rate of speaking and to physical proximity during normal conversation.

Shared Wisdom

"I find that substantiated, rehearsed responses to commonly asked questions not only promote one's professionalism but also promote the integrity of the entire massage therapy profession."

—*Greg St. Jacques, Director, Central Mass School of Massage and Therapy, Spencer, Massachusetts*

Non-Verbal Communication

Non-verbal cues, such as dress, posture, hygiene, and facial expression, sometimes communicate more clearly than words. While everyone would probably agree that a massage practitioner should dress and act professionally, opinions of what "professional" would look like are as diverse as are practitioners.

Dress and Hygiene

Good hygiene and proper attire are essential for anyone who works closely with others. Regarding attire, Diane Polseno addresses issues of dress in "Embody Ethics: Power Up Your Dress Code (Part One)" [*Massage Therapy Journal*, Winter 2001, pages 136-140]. In the 15 years she worked with or had been a client of massage therapists, she said she had seen everything from surgical scrubs to street clothes to shirts and ties. She saw a similar diversity in footwear. She wrote, "Each style that I have observed over the years has made a visual impression on me that could not be erased by what the therapist said, by what they knew, or by what their hands could do. When I received their work, if I was turned off by their appearance in any way, I found that I did not enjoy the massage experience, and I was not willing to seek their services again."

Similarly, posture, hygiene, and facial expression convey how you feel about yourself. They flavor the ambience of your practice as strongly as your words, policies, and techniques do. See chapter 6 for information about how your own self-care can add to your therapeutic relationship with the client.

One style will not attract or deter everyone. The issue of what is appropriate for you is dependent upon how well you know your clients and which clients you want to attract. What you wear and how you present yourself reflects your personal values and self-perception. Sometimes individuals undergo personal growth, maturity, and transformation over a period of years but still dress the same or react in the same ways, out of habit, that they always had. If you conduct a personal self-assessment regarding your own non-verbal image, you will have the opportunity to evaluate whether or not it is in keeping with your values and with your intended communication to clients. See "Dress and Hygiene Tips for Massage Therapists" (figure 5.2, page 199) for areas you might use as your checklist for maintaining appropriate dress and hygiene.

Figure 5.2   Dress and Hygiene Tips for Massage Therapists

- Your hair, body, and mouth should be clean and odor free.

- Pay specific attention to your hands. Because touching is the essence of massage therapy, clients will notice whether hands are clean and well groomed. Long fingernails could be a hazard. Keep fingernails short and well groomed.

- *Thorough handwashing before and after touching any client is an absolute must. Use warm water and antibacterial soap. Wash well with soap, in order to kill germs that are not eliminated by antibacterial cleansing gels. (For example, colds and flu are transmitted by viruses, not bacteria.)*

- *Avoid massaging any areas of a client's body where there is broken skin or a rash.*

- *If coughing or sneezing, either avoid client contact or wear a mask.*

- Massage therapy is physically demanding, so dress in comfortable clothing. White, because the color is associated with nurse's uniforms, conveys an image of professionalism. Some settings, such as healthcare facilities and spas, call for the use of uniform shirts and khaki pants.

- Keep changes of clothing at the workplace in case you perspire or get oil on your clothing.

- Clothing should be modest, to support your image as a professional. Be sure you are well covered when bending over. Avoid sleeveless outfits and short shorts.

- Shoes should provide support and be comfortable and neat. If you wear sandals, be sure your feet are clean and well groomed.

- Avoid wearing perfume or cologne.

- Avoid sharp, noisy, or dangling jewelry.

- Very long hair should be styled so as not to fall against clients.

   Source: Werner, Ruth, Trace Walton, Ben E. Benjamin. "Hygienic Methods for Massage Therapists." *Massage Therapy Journal*, Winter 1999, pages 24, 26-28, 31.

Note: Italicized tips above are required in the practice of standard precautions as defined by the Centers for Disease Control.

Presence Is a Form of Communication

The most gifted practitioners are present with the client in a way that is the very essence of good communication skills. Their whole selves are focused on the client and on the massage. To be totally present requires that you have a deep sense of self, of the client's mental and emotional state, and of the therapeutic connection between you and the client.

Ways of being fully present with the client include:
- Being on time for appointments
- Having the session room ready
- Listening with all your senses
- Maintaining eye contact

- Slowing down
- Single-pointed attention
- Attending exclusively to the client's needs

Shared Wisdom

"Be on time! Making clients wait gives them a bad impression before they even make it to the table!"

—*Laura Allen, The Whole You School of Massage & Bodywork, Rutherfordton, North Carolina*

In *The Educated Heart*, author Nina McIntosh writes about the ways in which practitioners may inadvertently burden the client with issues that detract from the client's needs. She writes:

Practitioners with good intentions can be misled by the notion that it's helpful to clients to be open with them about our personal issues. Actually, it can be a distraction in what is their time. What is really helpful to clients is giving them our full attention, and not dragging our personal lives into the session, or asking people who are paying us to also give us emotional support or free advice.

McIntosh writes that a remark as subtle as "I can't stand this hot weather," makes it sound to the client as though we're not up to par on a given day. Such a remark might interfere with the client's ability to trust the practitioner and fully derive benefit from that day's massage. To be fully present with the client is a skill that transcends minor errors of judgment or skill in other areas of communicating.

An Exercise to Help You Be Present with the Client

The following exercise can be helpful to you in learning to be aware of your stroke speed while staying present and mindful at the same time. Do this exercise with another practitioner who can give you knowledgeable feedback.

1. Warm up the back normally and get a good sense of the skin's warmth, texture, and color.
2. Increase your speed to a much faster than usual pace. Massage as quickly as you can without making your volunteer uncomfortable.
3. Note how you feel and sense how the client must feel. Go through similar observations detailed in step one.
4. Slow down. Go so slowly that you can barely see your hands move. Notice what is happening to the client's experience. What is happening to the space around you? How do you feel?
5. Stop. Stop right where you are and feel the skin beneath your hands. Go deeper. Feel the muscle tissue, the bones, and the viscera. Feel the blood moving and cells working to keep this body alive. Notice your fingers, palms, and the oil between the two surfaces. What does stopping feel like?
6. Come to a point between normal and fast, between normal and slow. Notice how the skin feels.
7. Return to your "normal" massage strokes, but this time experiment with different speeds. Know the difference between too fast and too slow.

Thich Nhat Hanh writes: "When we are capable of stopping, we begin to see and, if we can see, we understand." Once we master the ability to stop and notice, it will be possible to truly be with our clients and ourselves.

Source: Elizabeth Cornell. "How to Become a Better Therapist." *Massage Therapy Journal*, Summer 2001, pages 88-90, 92.

Multi-cultural Contexts

If a practitioner has more than one client, it's likely that he or she will experience working with multi-cultural aspects of therapeutic relationships with clients. In addition to cultural differences of clients from different countries, religions, and ethnicities, multi-cultural might also be construed to mean: age differences; attitudes (i.e., openness to alternative therapies); sexual orientation; language, physical, and economic differences; and victims of domestic violence, sexual abuse, or other trauma.

While it is outside the scope of this book to provide detailed information about working with each of the multi-cultural opportunities you might encounter, it will serve you well in all cases to let sensitivity to diversity be your guide. A sincere appreciation of all persons and a particular appreciation of differences are the main tools you need to excel in this area.

When You Go to Clients' Homes

A practitioner who provides massages to clients in their homes encounters many circumstances not found in office-based practices. In an office environment, the practitioner sets or abides by policies that are consistent for every client visit. When a practitioner goes into clients' homes, the practitioner must determine a set of practices and policies that will always be followed, as well as be flexible enough to adapt to each client's different environment. At no time should a practitioner alter his or her adherence to the code of ethics and standards of practice. The same standards of confidentiality, draping, hygiene, and client recordkeeping should be observed regardless of where the session takes place.

Beyond these core practices, the practitioner should decide how he or she wants to handle certain etiquette issues of being in someone else's home. Some practical considerations include the following:
- Ask the client where you should hang your coat or put your boots.
- Most clients will appreciate it if you remove your shoes at the door.
- Always request permission before using the rest room.

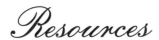

Information about Therapeutic Communications
- Cornell, Elizabeth. "How to Become a Better Therapist." *Massage Therapy Journal*, Summer 2001, pages 88-90, 92.
- Dunn, Teri, and Marian Williams. *Massage Therapy Guidelines for Hospital and Home Care, 4th Edition.* Information for People, Inc., 2001.
- McIntosh, Nina. *The Educated Heart.* Decatur Bainbridge Press, 1999.
- Nhat Hanh, Thich. *Peace Is Every Step.* New York: Bantam, 1992.

- Do not make comments on a client's furnishings or décor. You will be in the homes of clients who have more or less material goods, and any notice of their possessions could detract from the sense of therapeutic relationship you both desire.

When going to a client's home, sometimes called out-calls, the practitioner must be especially aware of security safeguards for personal safety. Make sure that someone knows where you will be, how to reach you there, and when you will return, and then let that person know when you have returned. When you enter the client's home, notice where exits are located and where you can reach a telephone.

Conflict Resolution

Conflict is a natural and even desirable feature of every professional's practice. Although it might sound like a negative term, it is in fact a normal occurrence in everyone's life and in everyday circumstances. It becomes negatively charged with emotion only when our response to it is ineffective. When conflict occurs, it offers an opportunity for the practitioner and the client to gain a clearer understanding of whatever topic is at issue. Conflict does not need to carry negative connotations; it holds the potential of illuminating information in such a way that leads to growth for all parties involved.

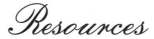

Support of Clients with Particular Needs
- Briere, John. *Child Abuse Trauma: Theory and Treatment of the Lasting Effects.* California: Sage Publications, 1992.
- Fitch, Pamela and Trish Dryden. "Recovering Body and Soul from Post-Traumatic Stress Disorder." *Massage Therapy Journal,* Spring 2000, pages 41-62.
- Matsakis, Aphrodite. *I Cannot Get Over It: A Handbook for Trauma Survivors.* California: Harbinger Press, 1996.
- McIntosh, Nina. *The Educated Heart.* Decatur Bainbridge Press, 1999.
- Persad, Randal S. *Massage Therapy Medications.* Toronto: Curties-Overzet Publications Inc., 2001.
- Redleaf, Angelica and Susan Baird. *Behind Closed Doors: Gender, Sexuality, and Touch in the Doctor/Patient Relationship.* Westport, CT: Auburn House, 1998.
- Timms, Robert and Patrick Connors. *Embodying Healing: Integrating Bodywork and Psychotherapy in Recovery from Childhood Sexual Abuse.* Vermont: Safer Society Press, 1992.

An important source of information is feedback from clients. How you will respond to the feedback determines whether it will help you. Here are some suggestions:

- First, be thankful for negative feedback. Most unhappy clients do not say anything; they just do not return. If you want to grow your practice, you will need to learn from your clients.
- Listen carefully, and take notes if possible. Listen not only to the words, but to the meaning behind the words. "That was an interesting massage!" can mean a lot of things. Ask specific questions to find out what the words mean.
- Stay centered. Focus on the needs of your client and your practice, instead of on your own disappointment with negative words, on your need for praise, or on making excuses. Avoid interrupting, and listen.
- When a client stops talking, use a process of reflecting, validating, and empathizing. Indicate your understanding with words such as "I see" or "I agree" or "You have a right to feel that way."
- Do not make excuses; they will not help you reach a solution.
- Discuss solutions with the client. Rather than telling the client what you cannot do, you will need to talk with him or her about what you can do to make things right.
- Tell the client what to expect, and then follow through on your promises.
- Thank the client for sharing constructive criticism or suggestions with you. If you learn from the experience and use it to help you grow your practice, your thanks will be sincere.

Source: Based on ideas in Hattie Bryant, *Small Business Today Guide to Beating the Odds: Expert Advice on Running a Business in Today's Competitive Climate.* Rocklin, CA: Prima Publishing, 1996.

Negotiation Skills

Negotiating isn't the same as arguing. When handled well, it is an opportunity for both parties to identify a solution that meets their needs. Here are some ways to negotiate successfully:

- Know what you want before you begin to negotiate.
- Stay centered. Remember that the professional with whom you are meeting needs clients, just as you need professional services. With this in mind, you can focus on reaching an agreement that suits you both.
- State your own needs as specifically and objectively as you can.
- Listen carefully to the other person. If the person says something you do not quite understand, ask for clarification.
- Restate what the other person says, using your own words. This can prevent misunderstandings.

Sending Clients to Others

At some time during your professional career, you may encounter a circumstance when it makes sense to suggest that a client change to another massage practitioner. Ultimately, your practice might be so busy that you will need to suggest that some of your clients try another practitioner. Or you may run across a client who may, for some reason, just be difficult for you to work with. If you are unable to resolve the difficulty, the success of your practice and your own well-being may require you to encourage clients to see other massage practitioners or professionals.

Building networks that help you build a larger client base by working with other massage practitioners and colleagues in allied professions is discussed in chapter 7. Building networks is an excellent marketing tool, and it is a strategy that serves a much broader purpose than encouraging clients to see others due to specific circumstances.

The following signs suggest it may be appropriate to ask the client to see another professional:

- The client (in the health history or other communication) alludes to a problem that is outside your scope of practice or beyond your skills. Suggest someone with the appropriate experience.
- The client does not like the technique you use.
- You find it difficult to maintain appropriate boundaries with the client. (For example, a mutual attraction is developing.)
- Despite your best efforts, the client always seems to be displeased with some aspect of the massage you provide.
- You instinctively have a bad feeling (fear, anger, revulsion) about providing a massage to the client. This person may need help from someone other than a massage practitioner.
- Part of your professional responsibility will include recognizing clients who have health problems that may affect whether or how you provide a massage. That's why it will be essential to obtain a health history when you see a client for the first time. Discussion of these conditions is beyond the scope of this book.

Whatever the cause, when you determine that you should suggest that the client see someone else, you should politely and clearly explain to the client the reason.

Providing Customer Service

Fortunately, most clients are delighted with massage and its many benefits. So you will be able to focus on the most important aspect of managing a practice, whether in your own office or at client sites: ensuring a high level of customer service. One survey of family practices conducted by Horizon Group Ltd. revealed that how a patient was greeted and helped by the support staff at a clinic was the number one influencer of patient satisfaction [Slater, Bill. "Reach Out and Touch Someone: Your Customer." *Alternative Healthcare Management*, January 2001, pages 25-27]. The article pointed out that even simple things like how to greet a client, how to respond to a client's inquiries, and how quickly you return a client's calls should be defined.

Customer service is as simple yet as complicated as knowing what your clients want and then providing that—plus a little more. Learning your clients' wants and needs will require a real commitment to listening to them and caring about them. You can listen and offer them choices every step of the way:

1. *Client inquiry*—When a client calls, ask about his or her needs. Would a particular modality or therapist be especially well suited for this client?
2. *Intake interview*—When a client arrives, have him or her complete an intake form (see chapter 3, figure 3.15 , page 142). Review it carefully and ask yourself: "Would the client benefit from modifications to my usual approach? Should the client be examined by a doctor before I begin?"
3. *Intake interview discussion*—Review the intake form and plan care with the client. Ask whether there are any areas the client does not want massaged. Review your policies with a first-time client.

4. *Feedback during the session*—Encourage the client to tell you what feels right and what does not during the session. Ask about positioning, discomfort, and use of oil. Adjust your approach accordingly. Many therapists use a scale of 1 to 5 or 1 to 10 to differentiate pain levels.

5. *Care after the session*—At the end of the session, ask the client, "How do you feel?" Summarize the session. Give appropriate suggestions, such as advice to drink plenty of water, stretch, rest, move, soak, and exercise. Also schedule the next session. A day later, call the client to ask how he or she is feeling.

6. *Referrals*—When a client has a condition requiring medical care, encourage him or her to see a doctor. If the condition involves skeletal alignment, you might suggest an appointment with a chiropractor.

7. *Suggestion box*—Provide a suggestion box and/or cards for client feedback. Regularly review suggestions, especially looking for themes, that is, related suggestions from several clients. Make changes accordingly.

8. Ask other health professionals if they have suggestions or expectations regarding your practice.

Be aware of the need to provide different kinds of support to first-time clients than to regularly established clients. You will want to spend an extra 15 minutes or so educating first-time clients on what to expect and on client intake information. If the client has had a massage before, but this is the first time with you, focus on how you can convert him or her to a loyal client. Regular monthly clients require an extra investment of your time as well, because they are the mainstay of your business. See chapter 7 for more information on how to gain new clients and retain existing ones.

You can enhance customer satisfaction by educating your clients about massage before, during, or after the session. Let them know what it can do. Likewise, be sure they understand what it cannot do. Massage provides many wonderful benefits, but it does not cure the common cold.

When you give the extras of good advice, suggestions for care, and responsiveness to concerns, you will find that your clients will return and will recommend you to their friends and colleagues. Satisfied clients will tell others about how your massage has helped them. The section "Client Self-Care Instruction" provides more detail about how you can help your clients improve their overall well-being.

Shared Wisdom
"Always be on time and prepared."

—Paula Curtiss, Healing Hands School, Pala Loma, Valley Center, California

Client Self-Care Instruction

Given the importance of a client taking responsibility for his or her own health, one of the most helpful things a practitioner can do for a client is to provide instruction on self-care. As a passive recipient, the client will not achieve the full benefits of active participation with the practitioner as a valued partner in achieving maximum well-being. It is important to honor the boundaries of the scope of practice for massage therapy within your state when you provide instruction on self-care to clients.

A program or routine of self-care may be focused on a particular goal, such as increasing range of motion, or more general, such as stress relief, personal growth, and general well-being. Self-care instruction to the client should incorporate awareness that established behavior patterns are difficult to change. Until self-care behavior becomes integrated into the client's daily routine, its benefits will not be fully achieved.

The most instructive action a practitioner can take is to model self-care behavior himself or herself. When a client observes the practitioner incorporating healthy practices in body mechanics, eating habits, attitude, exercise, and balance, the instruction is much more potent than oral or written instructions could ever be.

Techniques that can enhance the practitioner's effectiveness as an educator include the following:

1. *Use simplicity and repetition in spoken and written communication.*
   Give a client no more than three new pieces of information orally per session, and write brief instructions in simple terms. Include illustrations when possible. Accompany with demonstrations when applicable. Providing instructions on your office letterhead is more professional than scribbling a note on a scrap of paper. Ask the client to repeat the instructions back to you, to ensure that the explanation you gave was clear. This is especially important when working with clients for whom language-, learning-, or hearing impairments present challenges.

2. *Use demonstration, practice, feedback, and review.*
   Effective feedback involves auditory (rephrase or repeat the instructions), visual (demonstrate or show illustration), and kinesthetic (use hands-on corrective guidance) senses. At each session, acknowledge that learning new habits and ways of being in our bodies takes time and patience.

3. *Use social modeling to enhance learning.*
   The practitioner can be a powerful model to the client of the behaviors and level of body awareness needed. For areas of expertise outside of the massage practitioner's scope of practice, refer the client to high-quality instructional tapes or to reputable specialists.

4. *Gradually introduce the new behaviors.*
   A common mistake in providing client instruction is for the practitioner to forget that what seems commonplace to him or her may seem complex to the client. Clients are more successful in learning and continuing self-care practices if they are introduced to them gradually, increasing the number and complexity of actions as the client masters the previous ones. Clients are also more apt to stick with a program that is easily integrated into their daily routine.

5. *Give the client suggestions for creating environmental cues and modifications.*
   Cueing is the simple technique of adding reminders to the everyday environment, such as strategically placed reminders on notes placed on the bathroom mirror or the car's dashboard. Audio cues, such as clock set to chime at certain intervals, can also be helpful. Modifications a practitioner might suggest include installing an ergonomic mouse for the computer, buying an adjustable office chair, or turning off the television before the late-evening news.

6. *Encourage the client to use self-observation.*
   Self-observation entails taking the time to be focused and mindful of non-productive or self-defeating behaviors. Many people find keeping a journal helpful, as long as the recordkeeping itself does not become a source of stress or anxiety. Heightened attention through self-observation sheds light on habitual behaviors that were hidden from conscious awareness.

7. *Help the client create goals while focusing on the process.*
   After self-observation, the client may wish to write a goal or an action he or she will take to reach the goal. People who write down their goals, plans, and visions are significantly more likely to make progress toward achieving them. An important point to keep in mind is that a person's attention is best focused on the process of change and on removing the obstacles to change, rather than on straining for an immediate outcome.

8. *Help the client evaluate progress.*
   The practitioner can check in with the client periodically to help focus on how closely the client's behaviors match his or her intentions and how the client feels about the progress he or she is making.

9. *Provide positive reinforcement.*
   Self-care behaviors that involve a relatively long lag time between initiation and results put the client at risk for giving up. Creating external reinforcement to keep the client motivated until the intrinsic reinforcement (i.e., pain reduction) manifests itself is useful. The practitioner may provide positive comments and encouragement, and the client may ask a spouse, friend, or coworker to help provide supportive comments as well. Some clients enjoy making a contract with themselves to gain small rewards at milestones they set for themselves.

10. *Encourage behavior maintenance and social support.*
    At times of emotional stress, or when the client has an inadequate network of supportive people, he or she may relapse to old behaviors. If clients lack positive coping skills and a supportive social network, they may seek a level of emotional support from the practitioner that goes beyond professional boundaries. It may be appropriate to refer the client to specialized support groups, such as those for fibromyalgia, chronic fatigue, or cancer survivors. Practitioners will find it helpful to maintain a community resource directory and a referral list of competent professionals and organizations.

11. *Offer additional resources.*
    Provide information, such as articles or magazine subscription recommendations, names and addresses of alternative health centers, or notice of upcoming educational opportunities that the client might find helpful.

Adapted from "Strategies to Help Clients Practice Self-Care," by Patricia A. Sharpe. *Massage Therapy Journal*, Summer 2001, pages 50-62.

Ethics

In *The Educated Heart*, author Nina McIntosh writes, "Your relationship with the client is what will make or break your practice, much more than your knowledge of anatomy." Those relationships are based on communication skills, as discussed earlier in this chapter, and must be embedded within a firm context of professional ethics and standards.

Code of Ethics

Many professional organizations publish a code of ethics for their members to follow. Codes of ethics differ in the level of detail in which they describe ethical practices, but they all basically adhere to common attributes, as shown below.

Massage therapists shall:
1. Provide the highest quality massage therapy and serve the best interests of those who seek their professional services.
2. Respect each client's right to privacy and confidentiality.
3. Acknowledge individuals' inherent worth by not discriminating or behaving in any prejudicial manner with clients and/or colleagues.
4. Conduct all business activities within their scope of practice and the law.
5. Accept responsibility to do no harm to the physical, mental, and emotional well-being of self, clients, and associates.
6. Refrain from engaging in or tolerating any sexual conduct involving their clients.
7. Respect the rights of all ethical practitioners and cooperate with all health-care professionals in a friendly and professional manner.

Scope of Practice

Adherence to ethical standards requires that practitioners perform only those services that are sanctioned within the scope of their practice, as defined by their profession and by law.

It is critical that you understand your state's definition of the scope of practice for massage therapists, because violation of that scope would constitute breaking the law. Many states equate the functions of diagnosing, prescribing, and treating with practicing medicine, and they prohibit massage therapists from using such terms to describe their services. If you were to develop a marketing brochure and wrote that in your massage therapy practice you "treat" stress, you could be in violation of some states' laws.

Tipping—An Ethical Issue?

"Am I saying that massage therapists should accept tips? Certainly not. There are no rules when it comes to this complicated issue; although, I do think it is inappropriate for a massage therapist to solicit tips in any setting. What matters is that individual therapists have the right to determine for themselves, based on their clientele, their practice setting, their beliefs and their own appropriateness barometer, how to respond to a client who offers them a tip."

Source: Diane Polseno. "Ethically Speaking: Do You Accept Tips?" *Massage Therapy Journal*, Fall 2001, pages 148, 151.

Boundaries

It is important to have clear boundaries in the work setting. Boundaries refer to clear definitions of what you will do, what you will not do, and what you will accept and not accept in client behavior. Not only will you and your clients ultimately be most comfortable if you set boundaries, but it is your professional and ethical responsibility to do so. You will want to focus on the massage and whether it is providing the intended results. Massage can create a situation in which the client feels dependent on the massage therapist for enjoyment of the relaxation or pain relief.

Standards of Practice

Documented standards of practice help practitioners communicate clear guidelines to clients, which in turn helps clients understand and trust practitioners' boundaries. Such standards serve specific purposes, as follows:

- provide safe, consistent care
- determine the quality of care provided
- provide a common base to develop a practice
- support/preserve the basic rights of the client and professional massage therapist
- assist the public to understand what to expect from a professional massage therapist

Source: The American Massage Therapy Association's Standards of Practice

Shared Wisdom
"Teach students that this is a people business and the client comes first. Don't worry about how large a tip is—do your best, love what you do, and the rest will follow."

—Sister M. Janine Raphowski, Center for a Balanced Life, Inc., West St. Paul, Minnesota

Because these standards are specific, they are helpful to practitioners in determining appropriate professional boundaries. A few examples are shown below:

Shared Wisdom

"Be in touch with how you feel about people. People who have been bartenders and cocktail waitresses before becoming massage therapists do not have to go through the angst that others do—they've interacted with the public; they have learned tolerance for human frailty. Know your boundaries— what you can and cannot do and what you will and will not do."

—*Judy Dean, Agua Dulce Center and Spa, Prescott, Arizona*

Standard of Practice	*Example of Guideline*
Conduct of the practitioner	The practitioner seeks professional supervision or consultation consistent with promoting and maintaining appropriate application of skills and knowledge. (See "Supervision" section in chapter 8, page 291.)
Sanitation, hygiene, and safety	The practitioner maintains current knowledge and skills of pathophysiology and the appropriate application of massage.
Professional relationships with clients	The practitioner maintains appropriate professional standards of confidentiality.
Professional relationships with other professionals	The practitioner's referrals to other professionals are only made in the interest of the client.
Records	The practitioner establishes and maintains appropriate client records.
Marketing	The practitioner markets his/her practice in an accurate, truthful, and ethical manner.
Legal practice	The practitioner collaborates with all others practicing massage in a manner that is in compliance with national, state, or local municipal laws pertaining to the practice of professional massage.
Research	The practitioner doing research avoids financial or political relationships that may limit objectivity or create conflict of interest. (See "Research" section in chapter 8, page 283.)

Draping

Because of the close contact between client and practitioner, and the fact that the client is partially or fully unclothed, an innate degree of intimacy exists that distinguishes massage therapy from most other professions. Setting boundaries includes protecting the client's privacy with proper draping procedures, which strengthens the trust factor between client and practitioner.

For the first-time client, explain draping before the client goes into the session room. Let the client know that you will undrape only one part of the body at a time, as you are working on it. Let the client know that the genitals and female breasts will always be draped. The only exception is for breast massage, in which case the client will be asked to provide voluntary informed consent prior to the session. (See "Informed Consent" on page 214.)

Personal Safety and Security

Safety issues compound boundary issues when the massage therapist practices alone. As a professional, you are responsible for establishing a safe environment for both yourself and the client. Establishing such an environment involves three phases:

1. *Screening clients*—Whenever a new client calls for an appointment, request the person's name, day and evening phone numbers, referral source, and reason for calling. Then take a minute to explain the technique you use and what is expected of the client. This helps you identify callers who misunderstand the nature of massage. (If someone has misunderstood, remain calm and use this opportunity to educate people about the nature of the profession.) Before the client's appointment, call the number the client gave you, to verify that the client actually is at that number and to confirm the appointment time. Some practices have a policy of accepting only clients referred by a source they know. Others choose to clearly state to new clients before accepting an appointment that this is "nonsexual, therapeutic massage," to avoid possible misunderstanding.
2. *After the client arrives*—Have clients sign in or complete an intake form when they arrive. Take a few moments before beginning the session to establish why the client is there and what the client expects from the session. Then describe how you may be able to help the client.
3. *After the session begins*—If the client is uncomfortable with the therapy, you may choose to stop, and the client should not be responsible for payment. If you are uncomfortable with the client's behavior, you may cancel the session and request your fee.

Shared Wisdom

"1) Give your client your total attention for the time they are with you. Keep your boundaries clear and clean; 2) Don't use the little flower-shaped soaps in the bathroom when you make a home visit. They are only for show."

—Janis Legendre, IUPUI - Indiana University, Purdue University, Continuing Studies, Indianapolis, Indiana

Protecting Yourself When You Work Alone

- Make sure someone knows where you are, with whom, and when you will be finished.
- Work near a phone or have other means of calling for help. (Be sure to turn the telephone bell off or set it to low during sessions.)
- When you meet a client on-site, call someone (or even your answering machine) in the client's presence. State that you will be with the client (giving the client's name and address) and that you will call back after the session.
- If a client makes any inappropriate remark, state that it was inappropriate and end the session immediately. Ask the client to pay and leave.
- If you have to choose between staying safe and collecting your fee, stay safe.

Source: Cherie Sohnen-Moe. "Practice Management, Part I." *Massage Therapy Journal*, Fall 1997, pages 141-142, 144.

Dual Relationships

Within the context of performing massage therapy, the term *dual relationship* refers to situations in which two persons have a personal connection that goes beyond that of practitioner and client. The benefits of massage will be their most effective if the connection between the practitioner and the client is straightforward and uncluttered.

The best way to avoid dual relationships is to prevent them from developing. You should not encourage clients to discuss unrelated personal matters beyond light conversation. If, in spite of these precautions, you and the client decide you are drawn toward developing a personal relationship, you should refer the person to another practitioner. This helps to keep the boundary clear between the massage pracitioner's professional and personal life.

Advising and Counseling Clients

Staying within boundaries also applies to giving advice to clients. Practitioners would readily agree that giving advice on topics not related to massage therapy is strictly off-limits. The temptation to give advice in other areas, however, such as health care or spirituality might not be as easy to resist. Wanting to help others is intrinsic to the profession of massage therapy, and therefore it can be difficult to refrain from sharing with clients information that you feel would improve their lives in some way. Diane Polseno, in her *Ethically Speaking* column ["The Advice Trap," *Massage Therapy Journal*, Winter 2002], cited the following examples in which giving advice to clients exceeded the practitioners' scope of practice:

- A practitioner advised a client, who was seeing a chiropractor for lower-back problems, that he should "give massage a chance since massage therapy was less invasive." The client cancelled her next appointment with the chiropractor and explained her reason. The chiropractor took legal action against the practitioner for practicing medicine without a license.

- A client reported that she was taking antidepressants, and the practitioner recommended that the client experiment with an herbal antidepressant that the practitioner had found to be highly effective. The practitioner also told her that a specific pain the client had complained about could be a manifestation of the client's relationship issue with a parent. The client felt angry and violated and never returned for another visit.
- A practitioner who had devout spiritual beliefs and practices encouraged her clients to adopt a more spiritual lifestyle. She displayed spiritual literature in her office and offered to help clients learn how to pray and meditate for stress reduction. Clients soon sought out other massage practitioners and complained that they had felt pressured.
- A bodywork practitioner, who worked out regularly but had no formal education or credentials in personal or athletic training, offered his clients advice on how to strengthen muscles. One of his clients, who had an undiagnosed rotator cuff tendinitis, followed the practitioner's advice and as a result might need surgery.

In all these examples, the practitioner's intentions were to be helpful. But in all these examples, the practitioner went beyond the scope of practice and gave advice in areas for which he or she was not qualified or which were unrelated to the professional practice of massage therapy.

Some professional associations, such as the American Massage Therapy Association, provide a formal grievance process for members. Through this process, members can cite instances of alleged violation of the code of ethics, policy, or bylaws of the association. Violations could include such things as sexual misconduct, improper draping, and actions outside the massage therapist's scope of practice. The result of such a grievance, if the ensuing investigation proves that the violation did in fact occur, could be probation or suspension from the association's membership or expulsion from membership. The National Certification Board for Therapeutic Massage and Bodywork (NCBTMB) and many state regulatory agencies also have grievance processes.

Confidentiality

Confidentiality is one of the underlying tenets of the code of ethics for massage therapists. A client must feel confident that the information he or she shares with the practitioner will be kept in confidence unless the client expressly gives permission for that information to be shared with a designated other party, or the client's health is immediately compromised.

A confidentiality policy defines types of information that may not be disclosed to others without prior consent. The primary purpose of confidentiality policies is to protect your clients. Information about care should be shared—if the client signs a statement authorizing it—only with other professionals involved in the care and, if applicable, the insurance company paying the bill. Any other personal information clients choose to disclose during care should be strictly confidential (unless failure to disclose it would endanger someone). If you believe you must disclose information, be sure to discuss the situation with the appropriate person.

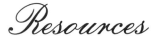

Information about Ethics and Boundaries

- Andrade, Carla-Krystin and Paul Clifford. *Outcome-Based Massage.* Lippincott Williams and Wilkins, 2001. See chapter 4, "Preparation and Positioning for Treatment," for thorough draping descriptions.
- Ashley, Martin. *Massage: A Career at Your Fingertips, 3rd Edition.* Enterprise Publishing, 1999. (See especially section III: Sex, Gender and Touch)
- Fritz, Sandy. *Mosby's Fundamentals of Therapeutic Massage, 2nd edition.* Mosby, 1999.
- McIntosh, Nina. *The Educated Heart.* Decatur Bainbridge Press, 1999.
- Polseno, Diane. "Ethically Speaking: The Advice Trap." *Massage Therapy Journal*, Winter 2002, pages 148-150.
- Polseno, Diane. Other "Ethically Speaking" columns in *Massage Therapy Journal*, 1998 through current issues.
- Redleaf, Angelica and Susan Baird. *Behind Closed Doors: Gender, Sexuality, and Touch in the Doctor/Patient Relationship.* Westport, CT: Auburn House, 1998.
- Taylor, Kylea. *The Ethics of Caring.* Santa Cruz, Calif.: Hanford Mead Publishers, 1995.

You can prevent some problems related to confidentiality by encouraging clients to disclose deeply personal matters to a trained counselor or psychologist, rather than to you. A massage therapist is not usually trained for counseling, nor is it within the massage therapist's scope of practice. Know your limits and be prepared to make referrals. Have a list of reputable counselors, psychologists, and psychiatrists on hand. Most clients will appreciate your caring and will respect the referral.

Informed Consent

The concept of informed consent originated in the 1960s, when the right of consumers to understand and agree to medical procedures became a nationally important topic known as patient's rights. Patients now must give consent for most medical care, except in emergency situations, and they also have the right to withhold or withdraw consent at any time. The concept of informed consent is now customary in many fields of health care. It holds the potential for reducing practitioner liability and litigation, because the client expressly consents to the services the massage therapist provides. But the value of informed consent is even greater if viewed as the foundation of an ethically safe experience for the client. See "Informed Consent Simplified Form" (chapter 3, figure 3.16, page 144) for more detail about the use of informed consent.

"Explaining Massage to a Client" (figure 5.3, below) offers ideas about how to keep clients well informed in your efforts to provide a more ethically safe and sound experience.

Figure 5.3   Explaining Massage to a Client

1. When new clients arrive for their appointments, introduce yourself with a firm, friendly handshake. Inform them that you are their massage therapist. Briefly describe your credentials as a qualified practitioner.
2. Use a client agreement form that eliminates any misunderstanding about what massage is and what it is not. (See chapter 3, page 144, for a sample form.)
3. Be aware of why the client is seeking massage. Ask the client at each pretreatment session what their goal is for the session. Meet their expectations if possible, or when it is not possible, explain why.
4. Assume nothing, and expect clients to assume nothing. Even if a client has received massage before, you do not know what that experience entailed. Tell the client what to expect during the session:
   - That most sessions are an hour in length, which means I will provide massage for 50 minutes and allow 10 minutes for undressing and dressing.
   - Remove as much clothing as you feel comfortable with.
   - I will use a high quality oil or lotion, but let me know if you are allergic to anything.
   - I will play music or work in silence. It's up to you.
   - To respect personal privacy, and for adequate warmth, I will cover or drape you with a sheet or towel so that only the part of the body being worked on is exposed at any given time.
   - Whether you want to talk or not depends on your need at the time. You are in charge of the session at all times.
5. Verbally inform clients what to expect by offering them a "Welcome" form to read after they fill out their medical history on the Client Intake Form.
6. During the massage, tell the client when you are moving to more vulnerable areas, such as the anterior neck, medial thigh, and abdomen.
7. Tell, or ask permission from, the client when you are about to rest your own body on the table, get up onto the table to assist your body mechanics, or to assist with stretches.
8. Tell the client when your work gets deeper, and check in to see if it is tolerable.
9. Inform the client five minutes before the massage is to end, and ask them if they would like you to move your focus to an area that may need more attention.
10. Perform tapotement only after explaining what it is and obtaining the client's permission. At the end of a relaxing treatment, it can be a startling experience to be awakened from a semi-sleep state to unexpected tapotement.
11. Don't surprise the client. Remember that information, knowledge, and the right to refuse offers personal power to the client who is in a vulnerable, relaxed state.
12. Inform the client about what to expect after the massage. For example, when suitable, tell the client that soreness or tenderness may be experienced the next day.
13. Cover all bases with your clients so that neither you nor they will face a situation without some preparedness. Let the only surprise be how much clients enjoyed the experience, and how impressed they were by your consideration and caring during the massage.

Adapted from "Ethically Speaking: Informed Consent," by Diane Polseno. *Massage Therapy Journal*, Spring 2001, pages 136-141.

Policy Setting

In chapter 2, you started to develop the fundamentals of your business plan. Part of that plan included the decisions you will make about the policies you will implement for your practice. Now that you have acquired more information about building a therapeutic relationship with your clients, and about ethics guidelines in the massage therapy profession, you have a stronger base upon which to make those decisions.

The "Policy Setting Worksheet" (figure 5.4, page 217) shows four categories in which your practice policies might be based: business, clients, employees, and professional development. The purpose of developing policies in each of these areas is not to become "policy heavy" in your business. Rather, considering each of these areas for potential policy development gives you the opportunity to decide whether a particular policy could help you set a solid foundation that could support a therapeutic relationship with your clients.

For instance, if your policy for clients arriving late to appointments says the client must pay for the full hour even if he or she arrived in time to receive only 20 minutes of massage, you would examine its effects on your business and on your clients. You would ask yourself such questions as:

- Would I enforce this policy even if I did not have another client in the next time slot?
- If a client did not agree with my policy, would I make an exception?
- If I did not have a policy about clients arriving late, what would be the effect on my business?
- Would I communicate this policy to clients before their first appointment so they would be aware of the importance of arriving on time?
- How would I instruct my employees to communicate this policy to clients?
- Would I post this policy on a sign in the reception area? Would I print it on my appointment cards?

Give particular thought to the questions about how you would communicate this policy to clients. Communicating policies could give you an opportunity to express your respect for all clients. Your explanation would include your commitment to policies that allow you to give full attention to each client.

You will need to go through a similar analysis of each of the policy areas shown on the worksheet. Try to anticipate the effect of each policy on your clients' willingness to continue making appointments with you. You will try to achieve a balance between the financial health of your business and your relationships with clients. Ultimately, if your practice follows policies that foster therapeutic relationships with clients, those relationships will help your practice grow and will benefit you financially.

Shared Wisdom

"Be sure to give each new client a check-up call one or two days after their first visit. This way you can answer any questions that have come up for them since their first massage with you. This is a courtesy call—you are not asking them to rebook an appointment with you. It shows you care."

—*Jocelyn Granger, Ann Arbor Institute of Massage Therapy, Ann Arbor, Michigan*

Figure 5.4

POLICY SETTING WORKSHEET

Page 1 of 2

Business Policies

1. Specify the code of ethics your business follows: _____
   _____

2. Specify the standards of practice your business follows: _____
   _____

3. We will accept clients during the following days/hours: _____

4. We charge clients according to (flat rate, any variations): _____
   _____

5. We will fully disclose our pricing structure to clients.

6. Our cancellation policy is: _____
   _____

7. Our late policy is: _____
   _____

8. We discount in the following instances: _____
   _____

9. We provide complimentary massage in the following instances: _____
   _____

10. We do/do not accept credit cards. Which ones? _____
    _____

11. We do/do not require payment in advance. Exceptions: _____
    _____

12. Our policies regarding safety and security are: _____
    _____
    _____

13. We do/do not allow the use of cell phones in our waiting area.

Client Policies

1. Our attitude toward customer service is: _____
   _____
   _____

2. Our policy for confidentiality with clients is: _____
   _____

3. We do/do not require an intake form with ❏ informed consent, ❏ medical authorization, and
   ❏ payment responsibility.

the
BUSINESS
of MASSAGE

© 2002 American Massage Therapy Association, Evanston, IL. *The Business of Massage.* All Rights Reserved. #20026

4. We do/do not require SOAP notes.

5. Our policy about boundaries between personal and professional relationships is: _____
_____
_____

6. Our policy about accepting new clients is: _____
_____

7. Our policy about referrals is: _____
_____

8. We do/do not accept insured clients.

Employee Policies

1. Employees' work hours and days are: _____
_____

2. Benefits paid to employees include: _____
_____

3. Dress and hygiene requirements are: _____
_____
_____

4. We do/do not allow employees to accept tips.

5. Our policy for confidentiality in communicating with employees is: _____
_____

6. Our policy regarding competition from employees is: _____
_____

7. Reasons to dismiss an employee are: _____
_____

8. Our policy on pay increases for employees is: _____
_____

Professional Development Policies

1. Our policy for communicating with colleagues and other healthcare professionals is: _____
_____

2. Our policy regarding taking continuing education is: _____
_____

the
BUSINESS
of MASSAGE

© 2002 American Massage Therapy Association, Evanston, IL. *The Business of Massage.* All Rights Reserved. #20026

Chapter Summary

The importance of establishing a therapeutic relationship with clients cannot be overstated. The term "therapeutic relationship" refers to a connection between you and the client that reflects ethical behaviors and codes of conduct, and sincerity and sensitivity in interpersonal communication skills. Your technical skills and your business skills might be excellent, but your business will suffer if you do not develop the ability to foster these strong relationships with your clients.

An understanding of the wellness model gives you a solid foundation on which to base your client relationships. The wellness model views health as the sum total of a person's environment, which includes mind and spirit, as well as body. This is in contrast to the allopathic, or medical, model, which is based on the concept that health is achieved through the removal of disease. Rather than focusing on the part of the body that appears to be ailing, the wellness approach focuses first on prevention and on examining the balance of all related components. Neither model is exclusive of the other, but they differ in the degree of emphasis placed on the physical body (the medical model) versus the integrated body, mind, and spirit (the wellness model).

Conveying to clients that you are supportive of their body, mind, and spiritual health, requires that you use good interpersonal communications skills. Good communication requires attention to verbal and non-verbal skills. Verbal skills include your choice of vocabulary and how you organize your thoughts, as well as your voice clarity, tone, and volume. Listening to clients and hearing what they mean as well as what they say is as important as delivering information to them.

Non-verbal factors that affect your communication with the client include your dress and hygiene, as well as the strength of your presence with the client. Presence includes such things as eye contact, slowing down, and giving all your attention to the client.

Professional tools, such as code of ethics and standards of practice, provide massage practicioners with specific guidelines on which to base their behavior. Letting your clients know the fundamental aspects of ethics and standards on which your practice is based helps establish immediate trust. These aspects include a broad range of confidentiality and boundary issues.

Creating policies for your business will give you the opportunity to anticipate how each policy could affect your therapeutic relationship with clients. It's important to keep a balance between policies that are client-friendly and also protect the financial health of your business. In the long-run, building relationships on trust and good communication will promote your business's growth while it yields the highest level of health and well-being to your clients.

Review Questions

1. What is the wellness model, and how is it different from the medical model?

2. Name at least three language skills that affect the quality of communicating with your clients.

3. What factors can cause a practitioner or a client not to listen effectively?

4. What non-verbal factors affect the quality of communicating with your clients?

5. In what instances might you find it necessary to suggest that a client see a different practitioner?

6. At what points in the client/therapist connection do you have an opportunity to provide customer service?

7. Why is it important to instruct the client in self-care?

8. What behaviors may a massage therapist demonstrate that are consistent with common healthcare professional ethics?

9. Name at least three areas in which adherence to boundaries is important to a massage therapist.

10. What is informed consent, and why is it important to the therapeutic relationship?

11. Name at least three policies you could establish for your practice that would influence the therapeutic relationship with your clients.

6

PRACTICING SELF-CARE

CHAPTER PREVIEW:

- Practitioner as Client Model

- Effects of Stress

- Self-Care Techniques

- Personal Self-Care Management Strategy

- Biomechanical Skills

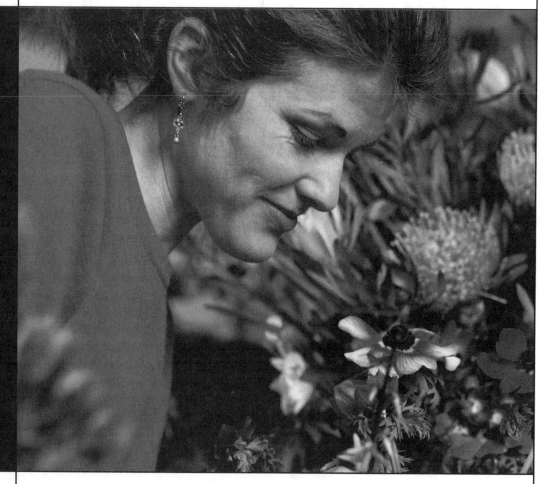

LEARN TO TAKE CARE OF YOURSELF AND YOU ACCOMPLISH THREE THINGS —YOU FEEL GREAT, YOU EXTEND THE LIFE OF YOUR PRACTICE, AND YOU GIVE YOUR CLIENTS A TERRIFIC ROLE MODEL. IT'S LIKE INSURANCE AND FREE ADVERTISING ROLLED INTO ONE!

Chapter Objectives

1. Identify physiological and psychological effects of stress.

2. Identify various stress reduction techniques and their benefits.

3. Identify strategies for stress management.

4. Identify strategies to prevent self-injury through the use of proper body mechanics and holistic methods.

Taking care of yourself is not only a critical requirement to operating your business, but also to establishing and maintaining healthy relationships with your clients. The content presented in this chapter is intended only to highlight the importance of self-care and to describe different approaches to integrating it into your business and daily life. Use the resources listed to expand ways in which you can effectively incorporate self-care into everything you do.

Practitioner As Client Model

Ralph Waldo Emerson, a famous U.S. philosopher and writer, wrote in the mid-1800s, "What you do speaks so loudly that I cannot hear what you say to the contrary." As chapter 5 points out, when a client observes you incorporating healthy practices in body mechanics, eating habits, attitude, exercise, and balance, your instructions to the client are much more potent than spoken instructions could ever be.

The principles of the wellness model (discussed in chapter 5) carry over into business practices as well as health practices. While most of this textbook focuses on skills and knowledge where the mind seems to be the most important—for instance, learning about licenses, taxes, and bookkeeping—the body and spirit aspects of running a business will equally influence the success of your business. If you don't take good care of your body, your longevity in the profession of massage therapy will be limited. And if you allow the daily challenges and frustrations of running a business to deplete your spiritual resources, you will diminish your creativity and your ability to communicate compassionately and clearly with clients and peers.

Effects of Stress

Massage practitioners are faced with not only the stress of running a business or managing a career, but they have the added stress of strenuous physical effort. Stress isn't necessarily a bad thing. It can motivate high levels of performance during peak periods of activity or during times of crisis. But if stress is prolonged and low-level, many parts of the mind, body, and spirit are affected negatively.

Physiological effects of chronic stress include high blood pressure (associated with heart disease and strokes), digestive problems, weight loss or gain, sleep disturbances, and memory or concentration problems.

Stress may affect you psychologically in the form of anxiety or depression. The effects of stress also diminish your general quality of life by reducing feelings of pleasure and accomplishment.

On the job, any of these stress-related outcomes will detract from the immediate pleasure of your massage career and also its long-term viability. Any steps you can take to diminish stress in your life will pay off in terms of satisfaction and effectiveness in your personal and business life.

Self-Care Techniques

Scheduling time for self-care helps you center yourself and reduce stress. Being centered or grounded means you feel a sense of purpose and are focused on that purpose. A sense of purpose can help you feel calm even in a stressful situation and competent even in a demanding situation. For many people, being centered also includes a feeling of being connected to a higher power. If this is a part of your belief system, it can be an enormous source of strength.

There are many ways to center oneself. The following methods have worked for others and may be helpful for you. Try these before, after, or during your working hours:
- meditating or praying
- using relaxation techniques
- walking quietly—a kind of meditation
- spending quiet time in a beautiful setting
- practicing breathwork
- practicing yoga

Try these outside your work:
- religion (attending a religion's worship services and practicing its teachings)
- reading books with spiritual messages
- support groups with people interested in spiritual development or related growth
- physical exercise
- sacred ritual (in a context you choose)
- keeping a spiritual journal, such as a dream journal or a gratitude journal (recording what you are thankful for each day)
- counseling with a spiritual adviser

Whichever techniques you choose, it is important to appreciate that the condition of being centered is not something you just decide to turn on like a light switch. Rather, it comes through ongoing spiritual and mental renewal, in a maturing process that continues over one's lifetime. If you are not used to tending to your mental and spiritual health, you may find that these methods seem awkward at first, and that the results come slowly. But continue to practice these techniques because they will help you make your career personally fulfilling as well as beneficial to your clients.

Don't overlook the importance of healthy physical care for yourself, which includes good nutrition and exercise. The most centered and grounded practitioner still needs to give the body necessary fuel to maintain a vigorous and demanding physical practice.

Get a Regular Massage

As you tell your clients and the public, massage can help both your body and your attitude. It can relieve stress and recharge your batteries. But if it is such a good thing, why do some massage therapists get so busy that they do not receive massages often enough themselves?

A central part of your self-care should be scheduling regular massages for yourself. This can be a great opportunity for barter. If you do not have enough cash to pay for a massage, you can trade services with another massage therapist.

Receiving a regular massage can also help with your professional development. Everyone has different areas of expertise, and you may pick up some techniques from the practitioner who provides your massage. In addition, you will be reminded of what it feels like to be the client. What can you learn about how you want to treat your clients? Indeed, there are several important reasons to regularly schedule time for your massage.

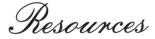

Links to Self-Care

- About Stress: http://stress.about.com (includes links to many helpful resources about stress management)
- Absolute Authority on Self-Care: www.absoluteauthority.com/Self_Care/ (a Web site with many links to stress management resources)
- Self-Care Connection: www.selfcareconnection.com (a personal coaching service with links to self-care resources)
- Stress Management Tips and Resources: www.stresstips.com (includes a self-assessment test on your level of stress)

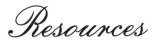

Information About Meditation and Spiritual Growth

- Through your religious organization
- Calvin, John. "Reverence Makes Bodywork More Meaningful." *Massage Therapy Journal*, Spring/Summer 1997.
- Cameron, Julia. *The Artist's Way: A Spiritual Path to Higher Creativity.* Tarcher/Perigree, 1992 (paperback, 1999).
- Crum, Thomas F. *Journey to Center: Lessons in Unifying Body, Mind, and Spirit.* New York: Fireside, 1997.
- Easwaran, Eknath. *Meditation.* Tomales, Calif.: Nilgiri Press, 1991. www.nilgiri.org
- Myss, Caroline. *Anatomy of the Spirit.* New York: Harmony Books, 1996.

Personal Self-Care Management Strategy

Scheduling your day is an essential work-related activity. A schedule becomes a tool for time management when you use it for all the activities you consider important. Some people are more comfortable adhering to a very well-defined schedule, such as one that says they will do 50 sit-ups every morning at 7:00 a.m. Others prefer a more loosely-defined schedule, such as saying they'll do 30 minutes of aerobic exercise three times a week. The point of building a schedule that includes work-related activities as well as self-care activities is that you consciously allocate time to a healthy balance of activities that help you and your business thrive.

Another helpful approach to self-care is to make it a regular topic of discussion with your mentor or your supervisor, if you use the practice of supervision. (See the section "Professional Growth Through Supervision" in chapter 8, page 291.)

Your schedule of integrated work and self-care practices might include time for many of the activities shown in "Practitioner Self-Care Checklist" (figure 6.1, page 226). Any items you check on this list should show up on your calendar. At first, it may seem odd to write "meditation" or "dinner with family" on your schedule, but aren't those activities as important to your life as the 60-minute massage you have scheduled to give this afternoon?

Biomechanical Skills

Besides receiving regular massages, you should take care of your body in other ways. Apply what you learned about body mechanics in your massage therapy training. Set aside time each day to rest your body. Take breaks to stretch your muscles. Get regular exercise, such as walking, hatha yoga, tai chi, or aerobics. Drink plenty of water and eat a healthful diet. Invest in office furniture that is designed ergonomically to be healthy for your body's comfort. These recommendations are wise for anyone; for someone in as physically demanding a career as massage therapy, they are essential.

Of particular concern to the massage therapist are repetitive strain injuries to the hands, wrists, arms, shoulders, and back. Most people have heard of the type of repetitive strain injury called carpal tunnel syndrome. This syndrome results from repeatedly putting too much pressure on a nerve that passes through the wrist, and symptoms include pain, tingling, numbness, and weakness of the wrist and hand.

Just as you advise your clients, if you begin to experience pain, numbness, and other possible symptoms of a repetitive strain injury, see your doctor and get a diagnosis. Follow the recommendations for treatment, which may include resting the affected area, stretching and flexing your muscles, ice therapy, massaging the affected area, and other means of physical rehabilitation. It is a good practice to pay attention to the way you work and to follow methods for preventing such problems.

Figure 6.1 PRACTITIONER SELF-CARE CHECKLIST

A schedule that regularly integrates self-care includes most of the following activities:

❑ Conducting massage sessions, including time to set up and get centered

❑ Keeping up with the paperwork of the practice

❑ Meeting regularly with my mentor

❑ Planning and tracking the progress of my practice

❑ Thinking of new ideas to market my practice

❑ Keeping my life fresh and interesting

❑ Continuing my education and training

❑ Networking

❑ Spending time with my children

❑ Spending time with my pets

❑ Spending time with my spouse, partner, or significant other

❑ Spending time with my friends

❑ Exercising

❑ Participating in sports

❑ Resting

❑ Taking vacations, traveling

❑ Meditating, reading, praying

❑ Taking part in hobbies, cultural activities, or other entertainment activities

❑ Participating in community, charity, and/or other religious organizations

❑ Doing volunteer work

❑ Other: _____

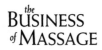

© 2002 American Massage Therapy Association, Evanston, IL. *The Business of Massage.* All Rights Reserved. #20026

Avoiding Repetitive Strain Injuries

- Warm up your body before you get started.
- Use the weight of your whole body; do not let your arms and shoulders do all the work.
- Use body mechanics principles, as well as stools and chairs that work for your body, allowing you to stay relaxed and comfortable.
- Keep the massage table at a comfortable height for your proper body mechanics.
- Do not wear yourself out. Schedule breaks, vary your activities, and limit your massage hours to what your body tells you it can handle.
- Use ice baths for your hands between massages.
- When a technique compromises you, choose another way.

Resources

Body Mechanics

- Andersen, Bob. "Stretching for the Massage Therapist," *Massage Therapy Journal*, Winter 1989.
- Butler, Sharon J. *Conquering Carpal Tunnel Syndrome and Other Repetitive Strain Injuries.* Oakland: New Harbinger, 1996.
- Fritz, Sandy. *Mosby's Fundamentals of Therapeutic Massage, 2nd Edition.* Mosby, 1999.
- Green, Lauriann. *Save Your Hands! Injury Prevention for Massage Therapists.* Seattle: Infinity Press, 1995.
- Machizuki, Sensei Shogo. *Hand Maintenance Guide for Massage Therapists*, text and video. 1-800-651-2662, www.japanesemassage.com
- Wolfe, Marian. *Body Mechanics and Self-Care Manual.* Upper Saddle River, N.J.: Prentice-Hall, 2001.

Shared Wisdom

"Continued education regarding body mechanics should be stressed to all students who are studying massage therapy. The correct use of body mechanics can help the longevity and successfulness of their business or career. It can make or break them. I've been practicing massage for over 25 years, and with the correct use of body mechanics, I am still going strong. Have a fellow massage therapist watch you as you give a massage."

—Sandy Fritz, Health Enrichment Center, Inc., Lapeer, MI

Chapter Summary

Practicing self-care is as important to your business success as your client and business skills are. A healthy self-care routine keeps your mind, body, and spirit prepared to do the demanding yet satisfying work required of massage therapists. Not only will your focus on self-care assist your own well-being, but it is a powerful tool as a role model to your clients.

Handling stress is one of the most significant self-care benefits. By learning processes to reduce or manage stress, you will minimize physiological effects such as high blood pressure and sleep disturbances, and psychological effects such as anxiety and depression. Techniques that can help you manage stress include meditation, spiritual/religious practices, breathing exercises, proper nutrition, regular exercise, and regular massages.

By scheduling these self-care techniques into your daily routine just as regularly as you schedule client appointments, you are taking care of yourself and your business at the same time.

Review Questions

1. What are some of the physiological and psychological effects of stress?

2. Identify various stress reduction techniques and their benefits.

3. Identify strategies for stress management.

4. Identify strategies to prevent self-injury through the use of proper body mechanics and holistic methods.

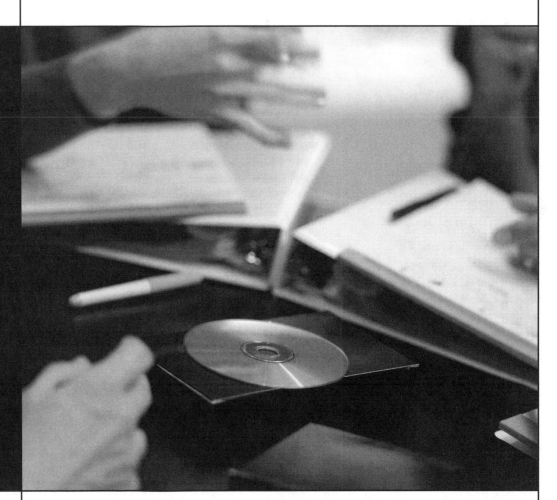

7 SPREADING *the* WORD

KNOWING HOW TO ATTRACT AND KEEP CLIENTS IS THE SECOND MOST IMPORTANT SKILL YOU WILL NEED TO RUN A PROFITABLE MASSAGE THERAPY BUSINESS. SOME WOULD SAY IT'S NUMBER ONE!

Chapter Objectives

1. Identify the four primary parts of a marketing plan.

2. Identify marketing strategies to develop and maintain a client base.

3. Describe tactics that are appropriate to each type of marketing strategy.

4. Identify the pros and cons of different marketing strategies.

5. Describe recovery strategies that you can implement if your business experiences a downturn.

The best technical and therapeutic skills in the world won't do you or others much good until you have clients coming through your door on a regular and repeated basis. Whether you enjoy the sales aspect of developing your practice or you see sales as a necessary evil, you will find that the right mix of effective marketing tools is the engine of your business.

Your Practice Identity

Every practice has its unique identity. In chapter 2, we discussed ways in which you would imprint an identity on your practice as an employee or as a business owner. In making decisions about launching your business, you determined a name that would convey a particular image. In chapter 3, we talked about building relationships with healthcare providers, particularly if you choose to accept insurance reimbursement clients. In chapter 4, we looked at various physical attributes (such as signage and convenient parking) that would attract clients to your business, and in chapter 5 we explored the therapeutic relationship you will establish with your clients. Now we take all these things that, combined, make up your practice identity, and learn how to communicate them effectively to attract and retain clients. This is the essence of marketing.

At the core of marketing is the concept being visible -easy to find and easy to reach. Actor and comedian Woody Allen's oft-quoted witticism that "80% of success is showing up" applies not just to scheduled appointments, but also to your general visibility to all prospective clients. You must decide how you will tell your potential clients about your services. Most massage therapists build their client base through a combination of referrals and a wide variety of marketing communication tactics and tools. For example, you can advertise in local newspapers and the business pages of a telephone directory, send a news release to the local paper, post signs near your target clients, or make presentations to community groups. Being listed in a print or online directory of massage therapists can be an excellent way for prospective clients to find you.

In order to use any of these tools effectively, you first need to develop a marketing plan.

Shared Wisdom

"Have a professional attitude at all times. When in public project an image that is positive. You never know when you will run into a present client (and everyone is a potential client), so be prepared with a positive, professional attitude—a smile and business cards."

—*Jeanne Troniao, Massage Training Institute of Bakersfield, Bakersfield, California*

Your Marketing Plan

Finding and keeping enough clients to make your practice successful is as simple — and as complex—as offering what people want, even exceeding their expectations, and making sure they know about it. You can reach people through marketing, which is simply all of the activities that go into developing, pricing, and distributing services and products and informing people about your services and products and their benefits. Let your imagination run free, and have fun. Marketing thrives on creativity.

In chapter 2 you were introduced to the "Career and Practice Planning Worksheet." In the marketing section, you were asked to describe your target clients, your products and services, your pricing, and communications. In this chapter we will explore principles and ideas that will allow you to flesh out in detail all the marketing steps that can breathe life into your business and keep it healthy.

Marketing Basics

Marketing is much more than advertising. In its simplest form, it represents activities for satisfying your clients' needs and wants. It includes planning, implementing, and evaluating the following marketing activities:

- Determining your market opportunities
- Selecting your target client categories
- Determining what services and/or goods to offer
- Setting prices
- Deciding where and when to offer services
- Planning how to communicate with your potential and current clients

An effective mix of these marketing activities will give you a good return on your marketing expenses. In other words, you will see an increase in income that more than offsets the cost of marketing. As you make marketing decisions concerning your practice, you may find it helpful to consider that marketing has long been used for many services. Indeed, history is a great teacher and can help you. To draw on experience, ask for help from your mentor and others with a massage therapy practice. Also do some basic research to read about others' marketing decisions:

The Small Business Administration publishes a variety of materials, including standard costs for types of marketing communications materials.

Professional publications, such as *Massage Therapy Journal* and *Massage Magazine*, include success stories in every issue. You can also pick up good tips and lessons from the letters to the editor departments in these publications. Read them and take note of the marketing decisions other successful therapists have made.

Check the marketing books in your local library to find anecdotes about successful companies. Take advantage of networking opportunities at professional association chapter meetings where you can gain excellent marketing guidance from your peers. Another way to connect with your peers is to participate in Web-site conference rooms, which are available on several sites. Other excellent sources of marketing ideas are your local chamber of commerce and business development organizations, which typically conduct marketing seminars and workshops for the benefit of local entrepreneurs. With a little imagination and creativity, you'll find that the same marketing ideas that work for other small businesses can work for a massage therapy business as well.

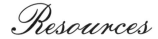

Where to Find More Ideas for Marketing Your Practice

- massage therapy Web site conference rooms, such as:
  American Massage Therapy Association: *www.amtamassage.org*
  Massage Therapy Web Central: *www.mtwc.com*
- your mentor
- professional associations' national, chapter, and regional meetings and conferences
- courses at your community college or at professional conferences
- Idea Café, The Small Business Gathering Place, at *www.ideacafe.com*
- articles in *Massage Therapy Journal* and *Massage Magazine*
- Cherie Sohnen-Moe, *Business Mastery, Third Edition* (Phoenix: Sohnen-Moe Associates, Inc., 1997)
- Martin Ashley, *Massage: A Career at Your Fingertips, Third Edition* (Enterprise Publishing, 1999)
- Terri Lonier, *Working Solo: The Real Guide to Freedom & Financial Success with Your Own Business, Second Edition* (New York: John Wiley & Sons, Inc., 1998)
- Jay Conrad Levinson, *Guerilla Marketing: Secrets for Making Big Profits from Your Small Business, Third Edition* (Boston: Houghton Mifflin Company, 1998)
- Anthony O. Putnam, *Marketing Your Services: A Step-by-Step Guide for Small Businesses and Professionals* (New York: John Wiley & Sons, Inc., 1990)
- Rick Crandall, *Marketing Your Services: For People Who Hate to Sell* (Lincolnwood, IL: NTC/Contemporary Publishing, 1996)

Marketing Goals, Strategies, Objectives, and Tactics

Applying marketing principles to your business efforts will help you reach your goals and objectives as a massage therapist. When you create a marketing plan, you will include four basic parts: 1) goals, 2) objectives, 3) strategies, and 4) tactics. Recall from chapter 2 that goals state your overall values and mission for your practice. Objectives are more specific, measurable statements of your goals. You can think of strategies as descriptions of how you will reach those goals. And tactics are actions that help you carry out your strategy. For each objective, you identify tactics, or actions, for carrying out the strategy. The following example illustrates these levels of planning:

Goal—overall values and mission
   Build a full-time practice.

Objective—specific and measurable statement of your goals
   Add five new wellness clients a month for ten months, until I am working more than half time.

Strategy—how you'll reach those goals

> Concentrate marketing efforts on health and fitness environments where prospective clients are most likely to be interested in health and wellness benefits.

Tactics—actions that help you carry out your strategy

> Offer seated chair massage demos at local health-food store, at which you distribute new-customer discount coupons. (See "Discounts: A Good Tactic?" on page 238.)

Write an informative article about the benefits of massage to be printed in your local fitness clubs' newsletters.

Give an educational presentation at your local fitness center.

Volunteer at local athletic or health fund-raiser event and distribute informative brochures and cards.

The reason goal-setting is your first step in making your marketing plan is that all other elements of the plan should be focused on achieving those goals.

Setting Your Goals

The goals you set when you begin your practice will focus primarily on generating a base of clients. Determining the total number of clients you intend to develop should balance with the number of hours you work per week, the demand for massage in your area, and your breakeven analysis. (See "Estimating Supply and Demand" section in chapter 2, pages 55-60). In addition, you should consider the modalities these clients will want. Typically, an established full-time practice requires about 105 total clients: 90 who make monthly appointments, eight to 10 to come in twice a month, and four or five who come in every week. Most massage therapists need two to three years to build a client base that size.

Setting Your Objectives

After you set your goals, your next step is to choose objectives that will help you achieve those goals. In what time frame do you want to achieve a specified and quantified result? Your goals will probably refer in some way to attracting and retaining clients. The more specific your objectives are, the easier it will be to create tactics that support them. For instance, the examples below refer to different ways to build your client base. By developing a separate objective in each category, it will be much easier to decide which tactics will work best than if your objective is too general.

Generating clients:

> How many new clients do I need or want (number and/or percentage growth)?

Cash versus insurance reimbursement:

> How many do I want as cash clients (direct access), and how many through insurance payments?

Focus of practice:

> Do I want new categories of clients?

Retaining clients:
> What percentage do I expect to retain as repeat clients? (Of course, you want most or all to come back, but 100 percent client retention is not realistic. What percentage do you retain, and do you want it to increase? If so, by how much?)

Increasing visit frequency:
> Are there clients who have expressed the desire to come on a regular basis, but don't? How many? How can you help them maintain a regularly scheduled massage appointment? What is the average increase of scheduled appointments by client per year? (A general rule is that clients should come monthly.) Be sensitive to clients' budgets and preferences. Recovering clients: If your goal is to expand your client base, how many former clients (number and/or percentage) do you want to bring back?

In answering these questions, you may want to develop different quantified objectives for different client categories.

Once you have created your goals and your objectives, you have a good foundation on which to make decisions about how you will go about fulfilling them. Your next step is to create a strategy.

Setting Your Strategy

Strategy refers to how you will achieve your goals. When you are starting your practice, reaching your goals will require marketing communication strategies for attracting clients. Most of these strategies involve learning what clients want and educating them about your services and how you can meet their needs. Your strategies will influence the types of marketing communications you will use. For instance, if you understand that referral networks are the major source of clients for massage, you will focus on developing them as one of your strongest marketing tools. Your strategy will also describe the appropriate balance of advertising and public relations tools. The following list contains brief descriptions of the types of marketing strategies you might choose from for your business:

- *Personal selling:* Face-to-face efforts to generate potential customers and encourage them to buy. Personal selling may occur at a meeting, a trade show, or anywhere you meet people. One form of personal selling is networking, also called referrals.
- *Advertising:* A paid form of communication in which the advertiser seeks to inform its audience and/or persuade the audience to act (for example, to buy something). Advertising may use a variety of media, including newspapers, magazines, yellow pages, radio, television, and the World Wide Web.
- *Public relations:* Nonpaid communication to influence opinions and beliefs. Methods of public relations include issuing news releases, holding news conferences and other public events, and participating in events likely to be covered by the news media.
- *Sales promotion:* Motivating offers to stimulate trials or increase demand. Examples include the use of gift certificates, discounts, and premiums.
- *Direct marketing:* Delivering a marketing message to and soliciting a response from individuals in a target market. Examples include telemarketing and direct-mail letters. In contrast to advertising and sales promotion, direct marketing is a personal form of communication. Examples include the telemarketer who calls your house asks for you individually and the letter that is addressed to you individually.

Comparative Strengths of Marketing Strategies

To carry out a strategy of, say, announcing the opening of your practice, you can combine referrals, advertising, public relations, and sales promotion marketing actions. Be aware of the type of response most likely to result from the following methods:

- Public relations builds general awareness of your practice.
- Networking and referrals build specific awareness of your practice.
- Advertising may be used for general awareness or to advertise a specific event.
- Sales promotion encourages people to make an appointment.

Thus, to encourage action as well as awareness, you need to create a variety of marketing communications tools. As you combine these tools, also keep in mind that they have different advantages and drawbacks:

- Referrals tend to take a long time to generate business. However, they will probably provide more clients than other marketing tools.
- Public relations costs less than other marketing communications, but the media—not you—control the final delivery of the message.
- Advertising costs more than other forms of communication, but it allows you to control the words used, as well as the placement and timing of the message.
- Sales promotion is intended to work quickly. It typically carries an expiration date (if expiration dates are allowed in the state or province in which you practice).

Another important part of strategy is choosing the audience—your target market—to whom you want to direct your message.

Your Target Market

The type of client you want to attract influences how you will market to them. The type of massage business you operate—medical, spa, wellness, fitness/sports, or specialty—will play a major role in who your targeted clients are. In the AMTA 2000 Market Segmentation Study, massage therapists identified the top three most important audiences to which to direct marketing and awareness messages as: 1) the medical community, 2) consumers, and 3) the news media.

The most important step you can take in choosing your target market is to know yourself. Reflect back on the "What Makes You Tick?" questions in chapter 1 (page 7), and think about your motivation to work, the things that are important to you, your ambitions, and the type of people you like to work around. Be clear about the things that give you satisfaction. Monica Roseberry, author of "Increase Your Clientele Through Mutual Marketing," described why she chose as her target market women between 25 and 75 who own their own businesses and are active in some way" (*Massage Magazine*, Sept/Oct. 1998). She wrote: "For my hands, women are easier to work on; for my head, entrepreneurs are more fun to talk to; for my heart, working women are a joy to help. For my finances, this niche market makes better money, has more flexible schedules, and, since my clients are both active and overworked, they have two rationally justifiable reasons for spending money on massage."

A more detailed answer to the "how" question that determines strategy is choosing which tactics you will use in carrying out your strategy. The next section describes a broad range of marketing practices and tools you can use to reach your target market.

Tactics—Marketing Practices

The type of tactics you choose will depend on what you're trying to achieve (your goals and objectives), and on your strategy for achieving them. Tactics are the actions you will take in order to achieve your goals.

Marketing practices could also be called tactics. They refer to the different ways in which you can gain visibility with your target market. You can see in "Marketing Practices Used by AMTA Members" figure 7.1, below) the types of marketing practices used by AMTA members. All of these practices can be effective, and it is your strategy that determines to what extent and at what time you want to employ any or all of them.

Figure 7.1 Marketing Practices Used by AMTA Members

Marketing Practice	Full-Time Therapists	Part-Time Therapists
Use printed business cards	94%	95%
Develop referral base among clients	79%	76%
Develop referral base among other professionals	66%	46%
Have printed brochures	61%	41%
Advertising (all types)	60%	37%
Advertise in yellow pages	49%	28%
Advertise in local newspapers	29%	18%
Advertise in local magazines	9%	4%
Advertise on local radio	7%	5%
Advertise on local TV	3%	1%
Advertise on other related Web sites	3%	1%
Display credentials	53%	41%
Use display signs	41%	28%
Speak at fairs	26%	16%
Issue press releases	18%	9%
Issue client newsletters	15%	9%
Use promotional items	13%	5%
Have a Web site for the practice	9%	2%
Direct mail/mailing	3%	1%
Volunteer or work at events	2%	2%
All other	13%	10%

Source: American Massage Therapy Association. *1998 General Membership Survey: Final Executive Report.*

Once you have selected the appropriate balance of marketing practices that fit your goals and your budget, you are ready to create the actual piece of advertising, or speech, or direct mail coupon that meets your needs. When you get to this stage, you will want to think in terms of which benefits are most likely to attract clients to your business. This is the concept of features and benefits.

Features and Benefits

When you are communicating with people about massage or about your practice, you can talk about their features and benefits:

Features are descriptions of the service itself—for example, how long is a session and what techniques does it involve?

Benefits describe the positive effects of receiving the service. They answer the question, What will it do for me? In general, when you want to get someone's interest or persuade someone to try something, you have to communicate the benefits along with the features.

"Sample Features and Benefits for a Massage Therapy Practice" (figure 7.2, below) provides examples of features and benefits related to a massage therapy practice. As you develop features and benefits for your own marketing communications, you will want to tie them back to your goals and objectives. Keeping a mental picture of your target market in mind as you work on features and benefits will be helpful.

Shared Wisdom

"Give incentives: Offer discounts like $10 off first session and give a 'punch card' where every 6th session is free. This gets the client in the door and keeps them coming. Sure, you will be doing a lot of free massages at times, but isn't that better than doing no massages!"

—*Laurie McCuistion, Licensed Massage Therapist, NCTMB, Magna, Utah*

[for another perspective on discounting, see "Discounts: A Good Tactic?" on page 238.]

Figure 7.2 Sample Features and Benefits for a Massage Therapy Practice

Features (Inform)	*Benefits* (Attract and Persuade)
One-hour or thirty-minute table massage or fifteen-minute chair massage.	Flexibility in scheduling sessions that fit your lifestyle.
Acupressure.	Relief of stress and muscle tension.
CDs and books on meditation available for sale.	Resources to help you relax between appointments.
Massage therapist is member of a professional association.	Assurance of quality care because therapist follows a professional code of ethics and standards of practice.
All therapists are licensed and nationally certified.	Confidence that care is provided by fully qualified professionals.

When you describe benefits that could attract targeted clients to your business, it will be helpful to be aware of the types of benefits that your clients might find appealing. Refer to "Benefits that Would Motivate Respondents to Have a Massage" (figure 7.3, page 238) to see what respondents to a 2001 survey said.

Figure 7.3 Benefits that Would Motivate Respondents to Have a Massage

The following are findings of a survey conducted by the Opinion Research Corporation, Princeton, New Jersey, and commissioned by the American Massage Therapy Association. The survey was conducted July 26-29, 2001, among a national probability sample of 1,000 adults (501 men and 499 women) ages 18 and older, living in private households in the continental United States. This survey has been conducted annually since June 1997. It is used here with permission from the American Massage Therapy Association.

Be aware that benefits that attract clients in your locale might differ from these national findings.

Type of Benefit	Percent of Respondents Naming Benefit
Medical Benefit	35%
Soreness/stiffness/spasm:	10%
Reduce/manage pain:	10%
Injury recovery and rehabilitation:	8%
Relaxation	15%
Stress reduction	10%
Pampering	31%
Other	10%

Percent = percent of survey respondents naming benefit

Discounts: A Good Tactic?

Most experienced massage therapists have strong opinions regarding whether discounting their services is a good marketing tactic or not. Both sides of the issue are shown below. Except in provinces that prohibit discounting, you will have to decide for yourself whether to include it among your marketing practices.

In Favor of Discounting
- a good promotional technique that could attract someone who has never tried massage before
- might attract clients who see massage as a luxury they cannot afford but who might become regular clients if they experience the benefits of one
- an expression of gratitude to regular clients, as in volume discounting
- might be considered a type of advertising expense if you use it to thank a client for referring a new client to you
- might be required as a condition of participating in an insurance company's or HMO's list of preferred providers
- could be valuable in promoting the profession in support of a cause, such as attracting attention to Breast Cancer Awareness Month or AMTA's National Massage Therapy Awareness Week™.

Opposed to Discounting
- massage is a health benefit, and health professionals do not offer their services at a discounted rate
- detracts from professionalism; i.e., dentists do not offer a bonus card for every 10th cleaning free
- an option to discounting that would not detract from professionalism is a sliding scale of fees to those in reduced financial circumstances
- some Canadian provinces prohibit discounting
- clients might come to expect discounts if they are offered too easily

Marketing Communications

Marketing communications involves telling people about the benefits of massage and how you can provide those benefits in a way that appeals to your clients' needs and interests. To do this, you can use printed materials, or electronic, or both.

Print Literature

Well-designed letterhead, envelopes, business cards, and postcards are excellent ways to communicate the benefits of your business. Types of print literature you might want to develop include the following:

- a brochure about the services your practice offers
- brochures about the benefits of massage—perhaps different brochures about different modalities or different client needs
- business cards on which one side contains your business information and the other can be used to note the date and time of the client's next appointment
- a price list
- notice of special offers or events
- notice offering gift certificates for special occasions
- cards requesting client feedback and suggestions

You may want to simply arrange these items on tables where clients will wait. Or you can place them in literature racks to keep them organized yet accessible. You might also use them as direct mail inserts.

Electronic Presence

Many practices, even very small ones, open a storefront on the Web in addition to their physical offices. When residents are seeking a massage therapist, they can ask friends for recommendations, call a professional association to get the names and numbers of local practitioners, look in the business pages of their local phone directory—or search on the Web. See the resources box, "Massage Therapy Directories," (page 240) for a list of some of the electronic directories already in existence. If prospective clients look on the Web, you want to be present!

You can be present on the Web in many ways. You can have your own Web site, on which you determine the extent of information and services you want to provide. Some practices simply have a home page that provides information about how to contact them. Others have extensive Web sites that allow them to schedule appointments electronically, order products online, take virtual tours of their practices, and access educational information. The choice of how much or how little information you choose to provide on your Web site will be determined by how much time you want to spend creating and updating the site, and how much money you want to spend.

You can extend your presence further by linking your site to other related sites, and to listing your practice with massage therapy directories.

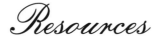

Massage Therapy Directories

The following Web sites provide electronic search capabilities to locate massage therapists. Make sure you're easy to find!

- AlternativeDr.com: www.alternativedr.com
- Associated Bodywork and Massage Professionals: www.abmp.com
- American Massage Therapy Association's Find a Massage Therapist®: www.amtamassage.org
- Dancing on the Path: www.dancingonthepath.com
- Holistic: www.holistic.com
- MassageNet: www.massagenet.com
- Massage Network: www.massagenetwork.com
- The Massage and Bodywork Resource Center: www.massageresource.com

Choosing Content for Your Web Site

Whether you produce content in-house or go to an outside provider, make sure the content of your Web site reflects your individual goals and that it's targeted to your audience. Other tips include:

- Check for spelling and grammatical errors, broken links, and other mistakes that can undermine your credibility.
- Make background information about your business available on the home page.
- Include a "last updated" message.
- Don't bog down your site with overlarge bandwidth-clogging graphics. Confronted with huge images that paint on their screen at glacial speed, many visitors will quickly move on to another site. One guideline is that no single graphic should be larger than 25 to 50 kilobytes.
- If you use clickable images as navigational tools, make sure you also include text-based links on the same page.
- Don't use colored or textured backgrounds that make text difficult to read. Likewise, dancing buttons, blinking text, and other bells and whistles can draw too much attention to themselves and detract from the overall effect.
- Don't link to unfinished pages or sections by showing an "Under Construction" sign. It's better to link to pages after you've completed them, preventing frustration when readers click for content they can't access.
- Always get permission for content you didn't create originally. *Getting Permission: How to License & Clear Copyrighted Materials Online & Off*, by Richard Stim, is a good resource to check for guidance in this area.

Adapted from *Personal Computing*, a syndicated column by Reid Goldsborough, author of *Straight Talk About the Information Superhighway*. Used by permission.

Choosing a Web Site Designer

A nationally syndicated technology columnist, Reid Goldsborough, offers the following guidelines when you first set up your Web site.

- Before you talk to anybody, clarify your goals for the site. Do you want to enhance your organization's image? Attract new customers? Sell products or services online?
- When talking with Web designers, ask to see a list of sites they've developed. Look critically at the designer's own Web site. Talk with the person who manages the sites the designer created.
- If you want to enhance or overhaul your existing site, first weed out outdated or extraneous material and then ask for a critique and an estimate from a designer.
- Don't meet with just the design firm's marketing people. Meet with the actual developers who will be doing the work.
- Ask about the consultant's or designer's range of expertise. Some may do just programming, some may also have marketing expertise. Some host sites as well as promote them, while others outsource to other service providers.
- Ask about arrangements for maintaining the site. A consultant can do this for you or provide the tools and training for you to do it in-house.
- Get an estimate of both time and money for completion of the site. It typically takes from several weeks to several months to build and test a site. If your designer works by the hour, request to be alerted if the project starts to go over budget.
- Make sure the consultant or designer you hire listens. Your site should be crafted to your specific needs, not a cookie-cutter of other sites. A good consultant asks as many questions as he answers.

Adapted from *Personal Computing*, a syndicated column by Reid Goldsborough, author of *Straight Talk About the Information Superhighway*. Used by permission.

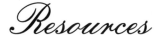

Information About Setting up a Web Site:

- your Internet service provider
- "An Internet Guide for Massage Therapists," *Massage Therapy Journal*, Winter 2001
- InterNIC (www.internic.net) - the site where you register your Web site
- Jim Sterne, "Even a Child Can Do It," *Inc. Technology* (June 15, 1999)
- your local computer store
- Massage 4 Life: www.massage4life.com
- Who Built It (http://www.whobuiltit.com) is a service that lets you type in an address of a Web site you really like and do find out who developed it. If it's one of the more than 10,000 listed, you can contact the developer.
- Aquent Partners (www.aquentpartners.com) is a temp agency that specializes in short-term Web work. It has offices in more than 40 cities across North America.

Many businesses make available on their Web sites copies of the same marketing communications literature they have available in print format. They also print their Web address on their literature, in order to gain the most efficiency from both print and electronic forms of media. Since it is faster and less expensive to provide frequently-changing information on a Web site than it is in print, many practices update their calendar of special events or promotions on their Web sites. They print in their brochures, "For our calendar of events and our special promotions, check our Web site at www ..."

Promotion and Advertising

Advertising

The greatest advantages of advertising are that it allows you to control your message and your business's image and to choose when and where that message will appear. You pay for advertising, so it's important to understand how to use it in a way that pays off. If your marketing tactics include developing and running advertisements, you must decide where to place the ads and whether to use display ads or classified ads. Because most massage therapy clients will come from your local area, advertising in the business directory pages (also known as yellow pages) or in publications serving the nearby community would most benefit you. See "Sample Business Directory Ad" (figure 7.4, page 243). Also consider whether you can buy ad space in publications serving the particular category of clients you are targeting. For example, use sports- or fitness-related newsletters or other publications if your target group is athletes. If your target group is performing artists, consider a dance newsletter.

Ultimately, the decisions about where to advertise depend on your knowledge of your clients. The better you get to know your target clients, the more information you will have for selecting where to advertise. See "Actions for Advertising Your Practice" (figure 7.5, page 244) for a list of ideas.

Despite its cost, advertising can contribute to a successful practice. Bob Waddington, who operates a massage center called Waddington's in the suburbs of Boston, regularly devotes ten percent of his gross income to advertising on radio and in the yellow pages, theater playbills, and newspapers. Waddington told Massage Therapy Journal (Mort Malkin, "Bob Waddington: Professionalism and Advertising," *Massage Therapy Journal*, Summer 1999, pages 96-100) that this strategy contributed to a 25 percent increase in gross revenue for two years running. His center, which employs twenty-five massage therapists, saw its revenues climb from $500,000 to $625,000.

Figure 7.4 SAMPLE BUSINESS DIRECTORY AD

ABC MASSAGE THERAPY, INC.
123 Any Street, Anywhere, USA - (555) 555-5555
Established in 1989

Each member of our staff is NCTMB, State Licensed,
an AMTA Professional Member, and trained in:

CranioSacral Therapy •
Myofascial Release •
Swedish Massage •
Reflexology •
Rolfing •
Shiatsu •
Trager •
Reiki •

We accept all major credit cards.
Massages given seven days a week by appointment.

the BUSINESS *of* MASSAGE

© 2002 American Massage Therapy Association, Evanston, IL. *The Business of Massage.* All Rights Reserved. #20026

Is Advertising Worth It?

Buying an ad that will reach a large audience can be quite an expensive way of communicating. In addition, it is by definition impersonal. The impersonal nature of advertising means that some people who see or hear the ad will not be interested in what you are offering. On the other hand, advertising is a way to reach people who might not otherwise think about massage or how it can benefit them.

You might try advertising for a short period and tracking the results. The simplest way is to ask each new client where he or she learned about your practice. Keep track of how much income you earn from clients who came as a result of your advertising. If the total income from these clients equals or exceeds the cost of the ads, the advertising makes business sense.

Figure 7.5   MARKETING ACTION IDEAS

Actions for Advertising Your Practice

❑ Post a sign outside your place of practice to identify it.

❑ Develop brochures about your practice.

❑ List your name in searchable directories on the Web.

❑ Become nationally certified by the National Certification Board for Therapeutic Massage and Bodywork (NCBTMB) and be listed on its referral service.

❑ Post signs inside your practice to announce special offers or new services.

❑ Place an advertisement in the business directory pages (sometimes known as *Yellow Pages*).

❑ Place an advertisement in your community's newspaper or weekly advertiser.

❑ Post oversized (postcard-sized) business cards on bulletin boards at health food stores, spas, salons, health clubs, etc.

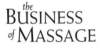

© 2002 American Massage Therapy Association, Evanston, IL. *The Business of Massage.* All Rights Reserved. #20026

Creating Effective Advertisements

Whether you design your own ads or pay someone else, you need to evaluate each ad idea to make sure it meets some basic criteria:

- What response do you want from the client after reading your ad (for example, calling to schedule an appointment)?
- Does your ad contain all the information a client needs in order to respond as you intend (name of your practice, phone number, location, and type of service being offered)?
- Does the ad clearly identify your credentials and the nature of your practice?
- Does the ad appeal to the client's needs and offer a way to meet those needs? (It should tell the benefits of your work as well as features of your practice.)
- Is the ad believable and truthful?
- Is the ad pleasing to see (or hear, for a radio ad)?
- Is the ad easy to understand? Test it on friends. Ask them to read or listen to it and tell you what it is asking people to do.

Sales Promotion

With sales promotion, you encourage appointments. For example, discount coupons cut the cost, so they reduce the perceived risk of trying a massage, thereby increasing the number of people who will make an appointment. For your reference in developing one, see "Sample Coupon" (figure 7.6, page 246). There are many possible coupon offers:

- first massage at 10 percent off
- free 10-minute chair massage
- pay for one session and get 50 percent off a session for a second person
- free merchandise with massage
- buy five massages, get one free
- discount of 50 percent off next visit for each new referral

In addition, there are many places to distribute coupons:

- health fairs
- newsletter for clients
- newsletter for target group (such as an employer or hobby group)
- at locations frequented by target groups (health clubs, hospitals)
- sports or dance events
- health-related businesses
- bulletin boards at client's place of work

Coded Coupons

When you distribute coupons to more than one group (for example, current and former clients, or at two different health fairs), be sure to code the coupons in some way. For example, you could give out yellow coupons at a track meet and blue coupons at a basketball tournament. Or, you could use a letter code to identify two-for-one offers versus a percentage discount. When the coupons are redeemed, keep track of their codes. This will help you decide which kinds of offers or places of distribution give the best results. When you evaluate your plan, you will be able to tell what is working and what is not.

Gift Certificates

You win in two ways when you sell a gift certificate. One, you get the money as soon as you sell the certificate, and two, often the recipient of the certificate is a new prospective client for you. Remember as you design or select your gift certificate format that you may be creating a first impression with its recipient. Be sure to convey the image you want for your business, and make the certificate as attractive and informative as possible.

A gift certificate should include the following information:
> The name of your business
> The address and phone number of your business
> Your business's regular working hours or "by appointment"
> An expiration date, *if one is allowed by law where you practice*

Optional messages, either printed on the certificate or in a separate note:
> Your business's philosophy
> The benefits of massage and bodywork
> Information about a particular modality if you specialize
> Inspirational quote
> A map with directions to your business
> Your business's marketing brochure

Shared Wisdom

"The single most important concept about advertising is that it should be cheap enough to be able to continue for a long time. Clients may see your ad running for months before responding to it. If the ad disappears quickly, they might think your business has failed."

—*Ian Kamm, Sutherland-Chan School and Teaching Clinic, Toronto, Ontario, Canada*

Figure 7.6

ABC MASSAGE THERAPY, INC.
123 Any Street, Anywhere, USA
(555) 555-5555

50% Coupon

**This coupon entitles you to
ONE FULL HOUR OF MASSAGE
for half (50%) the regular price!**

(must be redeemed by 12/31/03)

Ref. 09-A

50% Coupon

Note: Do not include an expiration date if not allowed by your state or province.

the BUSINESS *of* MASSAGE

© 2002 American Massage Therapy Association, Evanston, IL. *The Business of Massage.* All Rights Reserved. #20026

Shared Wisdom

"Reward your clients for doing your advertising. Offer them incentives for referring new clients to you. I give my clients a $5 gift certificate for each person they refer."

—Dori L. Facemyer, Oakes Massage Therapy College/Stark State College, Malvern, Ohio

Keep a log of gift certificates that shows who purchased them. If possible, also record the recipient's name, address, phone number, and whether the certificate was for a special occasion such as birthday or holiday. You can use this information to send future sales promotions or to make a follow-up call if the certificate is not redeemed quickly.

A caution about expiration dates: Some states and Canadian provinces prohibit the use of expiration dates on gift certificates. Be familiar with any laws that apply to you. If you practice in a state or province that allows you to use them, be flexible. If someone wants to use a certificate whose expiration date has passed, you will create goodwill if you accept it anyway. The potential long-term relationship with the certificate holder is almost certainly more valuable than your right to refuse the certificate. It's also up to you to let the certificate revert to the giver if it is not used by a certain date.

Cross-Promotion

As you develop professional relationships, you may find opportunities for cross promotion with others. This involves you and someone else agreeing on combined promotions that benefit both of you. For example, the health club from which you get regular referrals might advertise a half-price massage from you with every new membership. Those who are attracted to the club because of the promotion might become clients for you as well.

For a list of other sales promotion ideas, see "Actions for Sales Promotions" (figure 7.7, page 248).

Partnering with Other Businesses

I. Finding Small Businesses that Serve Your Market

Consider partnering in creative ways with other small businesses that are doing, or want to do, business with the same clients you're seeking. Take, for example, new mothers as prospective clients. What other businesses consider them clients?

Diaper services

Obstetricians/Gynecologists

Carpenters who specialize in room additions

Carpet cleaners who are getting the baby's room ready

Photographers who take baby portraits

Flower shops where the proud father will be buying a bouquet

Day-care centers that welcome babies

Stores that sell baby furniture, clothes, toys, baby books, strollers, etc.

II. Partnering with Small Businesses to Find New Clients

Level one: Acquire the business's customer list. You could buy it, ask for it as a favor, or trade massage for it.

Level two: Acquire the business's customer list, and ask the business for permission to use it as an endorser. The endorsement can be a quoted sentence or a letter written on your partner's business letterhead.

Level three: You create your own marketing materials, and the small business distributes them to its customers or displays them at its place of business. This can be as a favor, for massage, or for money.

Level four: You and your partner team up in joint advertising and marketing. Your partner promotes his or her product or service and uses massage as a reward for X number of repeat seals or X dollars spent. Massage could be awarded in the form of a gift certificate, discount coupon, or extra massage time with the purchase of an hour-long massage.

Level five: You and your partner team up again, but this time, instead of giving massage as the bonus, the reward is your partner's product or service when the customer buys X number of massages from you in some variation of a package deal. It's a reversal of level four. Businesses most likely to do this would be repeat services like hairdressers, personal trainers, and yoga teachers, or seasonal businesses like gardeners, golf pros and pool cleaners.

Adapted from: Monica Roseberry. "Increase Your Clientele Through Mutual Marketing." *Massage Magazine*, September/October 1998, pp. 53-59.

Figure 7.7

MARKETING ACTION IDEAS

Actions for Sales Promotions

❑ Mail your clients information about special offers (cheaper if you put a flyer or card into a bulk mailing from a direct-mail company; look for the company's phone number in the envelope the next time you get such a mailing).

❑ Provide discount coupons to target groups (potential clients or sources of referrals).

❑ Give discounts or premiums (such as a compact disc or a fifteen-minute chair massage) to clients who refer a friend or family member.

❑ Give away useful items with your name or logo imprinted on them (for example, pencils, combs, water bottles, refrigerator magnets) – especially useful to give to clients, whose friends may ask about the items.

❑ Offer a half-hour (or longer or shorter) massage in an auction for a community or charitable group.

❑ Have gift certificates available.

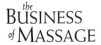

© 2002 American Massage Therapy Association, Evanston, IL. *The Business of Massage.* All Rights Reserved. #20026

Public Relations

Public relations generates awareness of your practice. It also enhances the positive image of massage and of your practice. Public relations could include actions such as issuing a news release, giving an educational talk to a community group, and volunteering at community outreach activities. When coupled with other types of marketing communications, public relations increases the likelihood that people will try a massage at your practice. The advantage of public relations is that it only costs your time and effort. The drawback is that you cannot control your message nor can you guarantee that your message will be publicized at all, in the case of a press release.

One of your greatest public relations assets could be membership in your professional association. When you are a member of a professional association that places high importance on educating the public and promoting the image of massage therapy, you can expect that the association will be an excellent resource for materials to help you better understand how to market and publicize your practice.

Among the tools you might expect are:
- a comprehensive and credible selection of research, published articles, methods and techniques, alternative and holistic care updates, and general information related to massage therapy
- easy-to-customize news releases
- reproducible fact sheets that provide information about such topics as: the efficacy of massage; consumer demand for massage therapy; statistics and attitudes of massage practitioners toward the profession; things you should know about working with health insurance reimbursements; information physicians should know about working with a massage therapist; and where to find research about the benefits of massage therapy
- presentation materials to simplify speaking engagements

You save time and money by becoming a member of a professional association that provides these benefits. These invaluable tools give you a solid groundwork on which to base your individualized public relations efforts to healthcare professionals and potential clients. The list shown in "Actions for Public Relations" (figure 7.8, below) offers ideas you can use to promote your business and your profession.

Figure 7.8

Actions for Public Relations

❑ Send out news releases to local media about your practice's opening (include information on your credentials and on the opening's date, time, and location).

❑ Send news releases about new services or new credentials.

❑ Set up a booth or table at community events, health fairs, county or state fairs.

❑ Participate in community outreach (such as the AMTA Massage Emergency Response Team™ in times of disaster).

❑ Join local community organizations for business professionals.

❑ Write articles for other businesses' newsletters (such as health clubs, medical practices, and wellness associations).

❑ Speak to a community group.

the
BUSINESS
of MASSAGE

© 2002 American Massage Therapy Association, Evanston, IL. *The Business of Massage.* All Rights Reserved. #20026

Figure 7.9

MARKETING ACTION IDEAS

Actions for Educating the Public

❏ Distribute educational brochures about massage and/or your practice at locations where people might be interested (health clinics, spas, health fairs, health food stores, recreation or park districts, community centers, libraries).

❏ Volunteer for AMTA chapter efforts to promote National Massage Therapy Awareness Week™ (This can give you opportunities to meet with the public and explain massage and its benefits.)

❏ Distribute preprinted brochures or newsletters about the benefits of massage therapy.

❏ Write to consumer media outlets to suggest feature story ideas.

❏ Suggest articles about massage for trade magazines, journals, and/or newsletters that provide information about complementary medicine, self-care, and health issues.

❏ Set up a Web site with information about your practice and the nature and benefits of massage.

❏ Give talks or demonstrations about massage benefits or your practice at health fairs, business meetings, recreation or park districts, or service or support organizations.

❏ Give complimentary on-site chair massage at community events, in stores, at malls, at sports events.

© 2002 American Massage Therapy Association, Evanston, IL. *The Business of Massage*. All Rights Reserved. #20026

Educating the Public About the Benefits of Massage

Massage therapy is still a relatively new concept to many people. Even those who have heard of "getting a massage" may not be quite sure about what it entails or how it might benefit them. Thus, a logical way to develop a client base is to educate the public.

Educating the public can involve giving talks or seminars or writing articles or news releases, if you think you might have a knack for any of these activities. If you do not like writing or public speaking, however, you still can provide information by setting up a booth at a health fair or distributing articles you have found informative. Whatever techniques you use, be sure your information explains the benefits of massage. "Actions for Educating the Public" (figure 7.9, above) contains a list of possibilities.

News Releases

If you have information that is newsworthy, it's possible that a local newspaper, magazine, radio or TV station would print or broadcast it. Attributes that make an item newsworthy include: it's educational, it's an *-est* of some sort (newest, largest, highest number), it's helpful, or it's timely.

When writing a news release, always include:
- your name and phone number where you can be reached
- headline that tells what's newsworthy
- dateline (gives city, state, and date)
- a paragraph or two that tell who, what, when, where, and why
- boilerplate information—gives reporters background information about your practice and other general but relevant information

See "Format for a News Release" (figure 7.10, page 252) and "Keeping Ties with Media Contacts" (below) for more information about successful news release placements.

Keeping Ties with Media Contacts

1. Develop a list of health, fitness and beauty editors, and reporters, and keep it current. As you develop a relationship with them, jot down notes about their preferences and interests.
2. Get to know the types of stories they cover, their deadlines, and how they work. Don't pitch stories to them that don't fit their criteria.
3. Invest in professional photos of your business's interior. Make sure the photos reflect the image you want to convey.
4. Have a fact sheet about your business on hand at all times, as a one-page reference to answer who, what, when, where and why. This is considered a backgrounder.
5. Regard any member of the press as your most hard-nosed critic. Pay close attention to how you package and deliver your information. You cannot control what they write. Return their calls and attend to their queries immediately. They are on constant deadline, and your response time will influence whether or not they use you for future stories.
6. Invite members of the press to try new modalities or services you offer. If possible, invite them to come with a friend so they can enjoy the experience more fully.
7. Designate yourself or someone else as a spokesperson. This person must be able to articulate expert advice on modalities, trends, and techniques.
8. Develop a "nose for news." Know what is news and what's not. Ask yourself why someone would care, and whether the information is either new, unusual, timely, or helpful in some way.
9. When your press release gets coverage, display clippings in your lobby. When you send out press information, include these clippings. It shows the editor that you're media worthy.
10. Public relations is far more effective with a personal touch. Remember editors and reporters on special occasions. Little gestures can make all the difference.

Adapted from "Are You Making the Most of Your Spa's Media Potential?" by Frederique Deleage, *Pulse*, May-June 2001.

Figure 7.10   FORMAT FOR NEWS RELEASE

For Immediate Release

Contact: [massage therapist's name]
                  [name of business]
                  [daytime telephone number]
                  [evening telephone number]

Name of Business
Announces ... [Event]

YOUR CITY/STATE/DATE – [NAME OF BUSINESS], a member of [name of professional association] [DESCRIBE ANNOUNCEMENT/EVENT].

[IN THIS NEXT PARAGRAPH, USE YOUR OWN WORDS AS A QUOTE THAT EXPLAINS OR ADDS COLOR TO THE INTRODUCTORY PARAGRAPH.]

[USE ALL OR PART OF A STANDARD OR "BOILERPLATE" STATEMENT. AMTA'S BOILERPLATE LANGUAGE IS SHOWN HERE] AMTA is a professional organization of 47,000 members. All AMTA Professional members have demonstrated a level of skill and knowledge through education and/or testing and are required to meet continuing education credits to retain membership. New professional members must be graduates of training programs accredited by the Commission on Massage Therapy Accreditation (COMTA), be graduates of AMTA Council of Schools member-schools, be Nationally Certified in Therapeutic Massage & Bodywork, or have a current AMTA-accepted city, state, or provincial license.

[ADD BOILERPLATE ABOUT YOUR BUSINESS.]

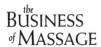

© 2002 American Massage Therapy Association, Evanston, IL. *The Business of Massage.* All Rights Reserved. #20026

Giving Speeches and Presentations

People who are not sure they want to pay for a massage may still be open to learning about massage or related topics. You can reach people with some level of interest by holding a seminar or workshop. Speeches help to generate awareness of your expertise and your practice. A well-delivered speech signals your professionalism that carries over into your practice.

When you accept a speaking engagement, choose a topic with which you are comfortable. Examples might be benefits of massage, massage of pregnant women or infants, or a particular modality. Prepare an outline and practice what you will say. Time yourself, and be sure to allow time for questions.

Know how to respond during a question-and-answer session if you do not know or are unsure of the answer to a question. Offer to take the person's name and phone number and call with the answer later. This is a great chance to follow up with someone interested in what you have to say. It also builds trust among the audience. Your audience sees that you give information only when you are sure of its accuracy.

For any type of presentation you give, take along plenty of business cards and brochures. People will pick up brochures on topics such as self-help. If your name and phone number are on the brochure, some of the audience members might call you later.

Shared Wisdom

"Do seated massage on TV talk shows and public access channels. It costs nothing, educates the public about massage and your business (people see who you are and what you do) and catches people's attention when they are channel surfing since most people have never seen a massage chair."

—Karen Craig, The Massage Institute of Memphis, Memphis, Tennessee

---

Resources

Materials for Handouts and Presentations

- American Massage Therapy Association, 820 Davis Street, Suite 100, Evanston, IL 60201-4444; (847) 864-0123; www.amtamassage.org
- Hemingway Massage Products; 815-877-5590; www.hemingwaymassageproducts.com
- Information for People, P.O. Box 1038, Olympia, WA 98507-1038; 800-754-9790 or (360) 754-9799; www.info4people.com
- Also see Resources: Sources of Preprinted Newsletters, page 262.

Publicizing Your Upcoming Presentation

You will want to do justice to your time in preparing your presentation by publicizing it in appropriate places, far enough in advance, to attract a suitable audience. The magazine *Alternative Health Management*, in its September 1999 issue, carried the following advice about how to publicize an upcoming presentation:

1. Publicize your event far enough in advance to meet publications' deadlines for calendars of events. These deadlines are usually earlier than most people realize.
2. Make up a few flyers and post them in your treatment rooms and lobby.
3. Tell all your clients.
4. Put up signs at health food stores and libraries.
5. Send news of your event to local papers and alternative health tabloids, and to local TV and radio stations.
6. At the event, ask attendees to sign up on your mailing list so you can notify them of future events.

Adapted from "Building the Business: Spreading the Word," by Lain Chroust Ehmann, *Alternative Health Management*, September 1999.

Massage Public Relations in Ohio

Jackie Stearns Jenkins, a massage therapist who practices in Ohio, is enthusiastic about marketing massage—and she has fun doing it. Jenkins and three of her colleagues took turns providing seated massages to the teachers at their children's schools.

The complimentary massages were a way to introduce the experience to people in a stressful profession, while thanking the teachers for their work with the children.

A few teachers who tried a massage signed on as clients. At the same time, the four massage therapists enjoyed the chance to visit one another and swap techniques.

On another occasion, Jenkins and two of the colleagues who visited the schools demonstrated massage to doctors at a local hospital. Many doctors were reluctant to take the printed materials or to spend time in a massage chair. However, those who did asked questions that signaled a definite interest in the potential of massage therapy. Besides giving demonstrations, Jenkins speaks about massage's benefits in various settings. In a hospital's cardiac-care classes, she teaches self-massage techniques as a form of stress reduction. She offers these services as a way to build appreciation for the profession, as well as to serve her community. Clearly, for Jenkins, marketing communications is an important business strategy.

Source: Jenkins, Jackie Stearns. "Thoughts on Promoting Massage." *Hands Across Ohio* (newsletter of AMTA Ohio Chapter). Fall 1998: 24.

Networking Systems

Most service businesses receive a large portion of their clients from recommendations—referrals from other professionals or word of mouth from satisfied clients. This strategy certainly applies to massage therapy. Many people are uncomfortable picking a name out of the yellow pages as a way to choose a massage therapist. The major ways of getting referrals are to use networking and personal selling.

When you are getting started, networking requires focused, concentrated effort. Your efforts at networking should encompass relationship-building with your clients, your colleagues, other business and professional people who may be sources of referrals, and groups that represent your target clients.

Networking starts with meeting people and letting them know what you do. Be prepared to present the benefits of massage. Be ready to answer the common query, "What do you do?" by developing a response that defines your practice in one minute or less. You might even plan how to demonstrate a few techniques that establish your credibility as a skilled massage therapist. You can introduce yourself in person, with a letter (such as "Sample Introduction Letter to Healthcare Practitioners" (see chapter 3, figure 3.24, page 158), or by asking your clients to refer their friends and making client referral cards available. (See "Sample Client Referral Card," figure 7.11, page 255.)

Figure 7.11 Sample Client Referral Card

ABC MASSAGE THERAPY, INC.
123 Any Atreet, Anywhere, USA (555) 555-5555

I, _____ , WAS REFERRED BY
        (new client name)

_____
            (referring client name)

Ref. 09-B

Massage therapists have an advantage over people in some other professions: people are generally curious about massage. When you introduce yourself as a massage therapist, many people immediately will have questions for you or be able to relate to the benefits you offer. Networking continues as people become acquainted with you and your practice and learn to appreciate your professionalism and other good qualities.

When you network successfully, people want your name and phone number so they can make an appointment or refer clients to you. Thus, it is important to have business cards and stationery that convey the desired image of your practice. See "Sample Business Card" (figure 7.12, below).

Figure 7.12 Sample Business Card

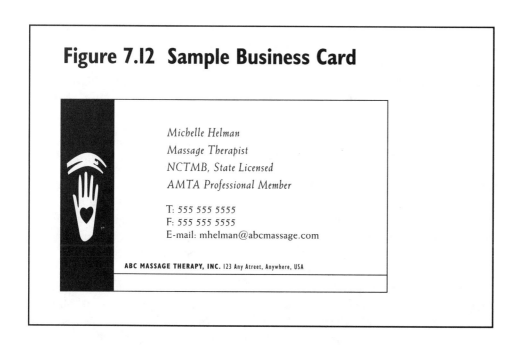

Michelle Helman
Massage Therapist
NCTMB, State Licensed
AMTA Professional Member

T: 555 555 5555
F: 555 555 5555
E-mail: mhelman@abcmassage.com

ABC MASSAGE THERAPY, INC. 123 Any Atreet, Anywhere, USA

Shared Wisdom

"To build a good referral base, start while you're a student. Your scope of practice is small and you will come across clients in need of psychotherapy, chiropractic, counseling, podiatry, dentistry, OB/Gyn, etc. Meet these professionals face to face and you will be able to build a referral base that will refer back to you."

—Kimberly Williams, Southeastern School of Neuromuscular & Massage Therapy, Inc, Charlotte, North Carolina

As you expand your practice, continue networking with clients and others. The longer you have been a massage therapist, the easier networking becomes, because your circle of acquaintances keeps expanding. Try to make a habit of meeting someone new every day.

People notice and care about whether those with whom they are networking are sincerely interested in them or just trying to get ahead. When you plan your networking, keep in mind all your usual ethical and etiquette standards.

Listen to others as well as promoting yourself. If you want to meet people by getting involved in a professional, charitable, or other organization, do it with sincerity and enthusiasm for the task at hand, as well as for the potential to promote yourself. When someone refers a client to you or praises your practice, be sure to thank the person, preferably in writing. Kindness always comes back. For additional ideas on how to promote your business using referrals and networking, see "Actions for Referrals" (figure 7.13, page 257).

Getting the Right Attitude

Teachers of sales skills agree that selling starts with attitude. You have to believe in yourself and in what you are selling. Here are some ways to arrive at that self-confidence:

- Reflect on what you learned in your massage therapy training and continuing education. What specific things were you taught? Which of them do you believe are helpful? Which are you especially good at? Imagine yourself doing those things, and reflect on how the client feels. Are you providing the client with something valuable?
- Reflect on massages you have received. How did you feel? How did it help you? Would someone else be able to benefit in similar ways? How do your skills compare with those of the practitioner you enjoyed the most?
- Reflect on what you know about the benefits of massage. Are you familiar with the efficacy studies on massage? Have you measured results, or have clients indicated positive change due to your care? What is your rationale for believing massage is beneficial? Would another person appreciate knowing about these potential benefits?

Whenever you have an opportunity to sell someone on the benefits of what you do, start from this understanding. You will be more confident if you remember that marketing massage does not mean convincing others to buy something they do not need; rather, you are enabling them to receive something that will contribute to their health and well-being.

Devise a 30-second "elevator speech" to describe what you do as a massage therapist. These short verbal explanations are called elevator speeches because they're the length of a short presentation you could give to someone during an elevator trip between floors. The ability to quickly and confidently present a sales message about your business will come in handy in many opportunities.

You also generate referrals by personal selling. Personal selling involves face-to-face interaction. Whenever you meet someone who might be a source of referrals, listen to that person, identify his or her needs, and explain how you can help him or her. You can choose your style of personal selling. The "soft sell" is probably best suited to massage therapists.

Figure 7.13

MARKETING ACTION IDEAS

Actions for Referrals

❑ Carry business cards and informational brochures with you wherever you go.

❑ Learn to say with pride and confidence that you are a massage therapist.

❑ Join professional organizations and business organizations, such as your chamber of commerce, local business association, and Better Business Bureau.

❑ Attend professional and business organization meetings regularly.

❑ Offer to present a talk or workshop to one of those groups.

❑ Actively participate in professional associations.

❑ Participate in breakfast clubs or similar networking groups. If one isn't available in your area, you might consider starting one.

❑ Participate in health fairs.

❑ Tell your doctor and other doctors you know about your practice and how it has helped clients; ask for referrals and indicate that you will refer clients to them.

❑ When clients express satisfaction with their progress, ask if you may write or speak to their physician about your practice and how it has helped them.

❑ Participate in or otherwise support groups that represent your target clients (for example, sports associations or track clubs if you want to target athletes; parenting groups if you want to emphasize prenatal or postnatal care or infant massage; social organizations or support groups if you want to target people in the relevant categories).

❑ Send letters to healthcare professionals, requesting referrals.

❑ Always send a thank you for a referral, even if the person referred to you doesn't make an appointment.

the
BUSINESS
of MASSAGE

© 2002 American Massage Therapy Association, Evanston, IL. *The Business of Massage.* All Rights Reserved. #20026

Although some people associate selling with talking, you will be most effective if you listen well. When others talk, listen for the needs they express. If you see how your practice can help with those needs, you can offer a solution. People appreciate being convinced when its aim is to help them.

Responsibilities and Liabilities

It is important that you take special care in your oral and written communications with clients and other professionals that you accept the full responsibility of your professional status as a massage practitioner. This means adhering to the scope of practice, the code of ethics, and all regulations that apply to you in your state or province. Make sure you have a client's signed release of information (see chapter 3, figure 3.17, page 145.) before sending client records to another practitioner or clinician who has been specified by name on the client's release form.

Also be especially sensitive to your use of terminology in communicating in writing and orally. Since "treatment" is outside the scope of practice for massage practitioners in many states, be careful not to use the term even in ways that seem generic to you, such as "treating" a client for stress.

Attracting Clients at Stages of Business

Building Your Client Base

Once you have announced your practice's opening, you will want to build on that communication. You can do this by using all of the strategies discussed previously in this chapter: personal selling (networking and referrals), advertising, public relations, sales promotion, and direct marketing.

The strategies you choose will depend on the type of business you start, your target market, and your budget. General steps you will modify to suit your own business include:

1. Become familiar with the individuals and organizations most likely to share common interests with your business goals.
2. Introduce yourself to individuals and organizations whose members or client groups might also be clients of yours.
3. Choose a mix of strategies designed to achieve short-term results as well as long-term growth. For instance, advertising and sales promotions provide the fastest results, even though they are among the more expensive strategies. Public relations activities are aimed at longer-term visibility and education.
4. Once you have chosen appropriate strategies, refer to the "Marketing Action Ideas" throughout this chapter for ideas about specific tactics to use.

For an example of how one massage therapist has been successful in seeking clients, see "Tips on How to Seek Clients in a Wellness Setting" on page 259.

Tips on How to Seek Clients in a Wellness Setting

Marilyn Kier, AMTA professional member and massage therapist/owner of Wellness at Work, in Northfield, Illinois, specializes in providing on-site seated massage to employees in wellness programs at companies like Motorola, Discover Financial Services, and a local two-year college. She offers the following tips on how to seek clients in a wellness setting:

1. Get to Know Wellness Professionals/Let Them Get to Know You
   - Become active in your local chapter of Wellness Councils of America.
   - Attend national or regional conferences of the Association of Worksite Health Promotion (AWHP).
   - Join the local chamber of commerce.
   - Give talks to organizations on topics such as ergonomics, relaxation, and different types of massage.
   - At a company, the person who handles wellness benefits might be a director of wellness, a director of work and family benefits, or a human resources director.
   - At a hospital, first distinguish between wellness programs for patients and wellness programs for employees or staff. There might be a wellness committee, directed by Human Resources. Many hospitals have or are developing community-based wellness centers for integrated care.
   - At a university or college, the staff/faculty wellness program might reside in a Department of Health & Psychological Services, and be headed by a wellness coordinator.

2. Introduce Yourself
   - When you have a contact person's name, send that person and letter and then follow up with a phone call and request an appointment to talk about how you could help. In the appointment, give a demonstration of your services.
   - Initial questions to ask: Do you have a wellness program? Are you thinking of implementing one? Are you familiar with seated massage?

3. Negotiate a Profitable Working Relationship
   - Employee participation is higher if the company's budget pays for them to receive on-site seated massages, vs. if the employee pays partial costs.
   - Suggest the company pay you by the hour rather than by the massage, because you will have transition times between massages that are otherwise unpaid.

4. Conduct Your On-site Business Professionally
   - Plan for three 15-minute massages per hour. You need five minutes between massages to sanitize the chair after previous client, greet the new client, establish rapport, ask questions about contraindications, and adjust the chair.
   - It's important to be efficient without conveying an assembly-line approach.
   - Be a role model for self-care. If you work a seven-hour day—that's 21 clients a day—make sure to take necessary breaks, drink fluids, and use proper biomechanical posture and movements.

5. Find out if companies' health plans include flex benefits, and if employees can use their pre-tax flex benefits for massage therapy and bodywork.
   - If so, ask how you can communicate that fact to employees.
   - Find out when the flex benefit account is closed out each year, and send a notice to employees two months before to remind them how they can prevent those benefits from going to waste.

Source: "Practice-Building Tips: Working in Medical and Wellness Settings." ©2001 American Massage Therapy Association.

Retaining Clients

According to the U.S. Chamber of Commerce, keeping clients is easier than winning new ones. That is why an important goal for massage therapists is to keep your clients coming back. You can do this by encouraging ongoing client relationships and bringing back your former clients.

Encouraging Ongoing Client Relationships

Clients keep coming back when they feel they have a professional, beneficial relationship with you. Therefore, efforts to encourage ongoing client relationships often are called "relationship marketing." Relationship marketing includes all the ways you strengthen your professional ties with clients, including client education and follow-up.

Relationship marketing requires the best of personal selling methods: listening to clients, taking notes, and carefully assessing clients' needs. At the end of each session, evaluate the client's situation. Encourage the use of other therapies and products if you believe they will enhance the client's well-being.

Staying in Touch with Clients

Chances are, many clients do not fully appreciate all the ways they can benefit from the services and products your practice offers. Thus, you can foster ongoing relationships through education of your clients. Remember that education is a long-term process, one that needs constant attention.

Many practitioners conduct what they call "exit interviews," particularly after a client's first session, in which they ask about the client's experience and satisfaction. Even if you conduct such an interview, some clients will not come back unless you follow up with them. Client follow-up is a good way to demonstrate that you care about your clients and want them to have a positive experience with your practice. It also shows that you follow through with the care plan, including return visits.

Remember, it is much easier and less expensive to keep your existing clients coming back than it is to attract new clients. It is your existing clients who already know about you and about massage. After yourself, repeat clients are your practice's most valued resource. Not only do you have their business, but they can be your best source of referrals. By providing your existing clients with a consistently high level of service and care, you allow them to trust that anyone they refer also will be pleased.

See "Actions for Client Retention" (figure 7.14, page 261) and "Actions for Staying in Touch" (figure 7.15, page 262) for suggested ideas about how to keep your clients once you've attracted them to an initial appointment.

Shared Wisdom

Evaluate your return client percentage. If 50% or less of your clients do not schedule an appointment within three months it is time to consider taking a business strategies course.

—*Van Delia, Onandaga School of Therapeutic Massage, Syracuse, New York*

Figure 7.14

MARKETING ACTION IDEAS

Actions for Client Retention

❏ Before the appointment, call the client or send a reminder postcard with a reminder of the appointment day and time.

❏ Increase the likelihood that clients will evaluate their experience in a positive way by discussing their situation and expectations before the session begins. Learn whether clients have reasonable expectations.

❏ Vary your techniques and style. If you give the same massage every time, it will become repetitive.

❏ Take courses in new modalities and techniques from time to time, to keep your work and style fresh to clients.

❏ Learn about the client's life habits before the session begins. This will help you tailor your service to each client's needs.

❏ Provide a level of service that makes clients feel nurtured – promptness at appointments, clear explanations, a glass of water, a warm washcloth for wiping off oil.

❏ Focus completely on the client when in session. At the end of the session, conduct an exit interview to gather information about the client's impressions of the session. (This can help the client notice such benefits as relaxed muscles or reduced pain.)

❏ Formulate a care plan utilizing formal records such as SOAP notes to help you and the client increase progress.

❏ Tell clients about the benefits they can receive if they visit more often.

❏ Teach self-care measures for clients to use at home between visits.

❏ Before clients leave, encourage them to book their next appointment(s). For example, say, "You are in great shape. Once a month would really make a difference for you," or, "Until you are out of the acute pain, let's do twice per week for several weeks. Then we can re-evaluate the situation and maybe move to once a week." Some therapists have their clients sign up for a year in advance. Some clients with busy schedules like the idea that, routinely, the day and time are committed for massage. Others will feel that setting a regular time is restrictive and will prefer to schedule each session individually.

❏ Provide literature about massage and any other services offered by your practice for clients to take home or read while waiting for their appointment.

❏ Offer special packages for clients, such as discounts for a series of three, five, or ten massages; a tenth massage at no charge; or a free session after a client has brought in five referrals.

❏ Consider collaborating with other alternative health professionals and offering a lecture series.

❏ In a prominent place, display a card saying, "Our business continues to grow through your referrals. Thank you for recommending us."

❏ Always send an individual thank-you card for referrals.

the
BUSINESS
of MASSAGE

© 2002 American Massage Therapy Association, Evanston, IL. *The Business of Massage.* All Rights Reserved. #20026

Figure 7.15

MARKETING ACTION IDEAS

Actions for Staying in Touch

❑ One day to two weeks after each appointment, call clients to ask how they are doing. Ask them if they are drinking enough water, doing suggested exercises, or following any other advice you discussed in their exit interview.

❑ Send clients copies of magazine or newspaper articles or the results of new research on aspects of massage related to their needs.

❑ Call to remind clients of their next appointment or to make their next appointment.

❑ Send clients newsletters, postcards, or flyers to tell them about specials, new services, or new pricing.

❑ Send cards on clients' birthdays or around special occasions such as Mother's Day, Valentine's Day, or even ski season – whatever will be relevant to your targeted client type.

❑ Give clients an opportunity to answer short questionnaires about their satisfaction with the massage and their overall experience with your practice.

❑ Host special events for clients at your practice, honoring, for example, AMTA's National Massage Therapy Awareness Week or the anniversary of your practice.

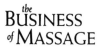

© 2002 American Massage Therapy Association, Evanston, IL. *The Business of Massage.* All Rights Reserved. #20026

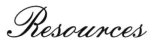

Sources of Preprinted Newsletters

- Collier Communications (www.colliercom.com)
- *Food for Thought Health News,* 727-446-8405
- *Healing Ink,* 4938 Hampden Lane, Bethesda, MD 20814, 1-888-558-2747, healingink@msn.com
- *Staying in Touch,* 877-634-1010, www.stayingintouch.net
- *TopHealth: The Health Promotion and Wellness Letter* (www.toptopics.com)

Through your marketing communications, your clients will form an impression about you and your practice. But no matter what marketing communications techniques you use, remember that the most important element of marketing your practice is yourself. People will respond to your skill, your professionalism, your enthusiasm, and your concern for their well-being. Do what it takes to project a positive, caring attitude, and clients will keep coming back for more.

Growing Your Practice

What makes a massage therapy practice grow? It is a combination of you, your practice, and your clients. When you want your practice to grow, take some time to review how far you have come and decide how to build on what you have learned. You may decide to move from part-time to full-time, add services and products, specialize, hire employees, or pursue related opportunities such as teaching or research. Apply the ideas in this manual and the counsel of others to make your vision of a growing practice come true.

Growth Strategies

When you decide you are ready to nurture growth in your practice, decide what combination of strategies is right for you. Among basic growth strategies are to move from part-time to full-time, to diversify your current offerings, or to specialize.

In developing such a growth strategy, it is important to understand what "part-time" and "full-time" mean for a massage therapist. Massage is physically hard work. No one can be expected to spend 40 hours a week providing massages. Rather, a full-time massage therapist has been self-defined by AMTA members as someone who provides 17-or-more paid massage hours per week. In addition, this person devotes other hours during the week to client follow-up, education of self and others, managing the practice, and so on.

There are a variety of service tactics for expanding into a full-time practice:
- Rent an office if you have not already done so.
- Increase your number of massage hours (setting up office hours and planning to be there to accept walk-ins).
- Hire massage staff—employees or independent contractors—to expand the massage hours you offer or locations at which you work.
- Hire support staff to help with phone calls and paperwork.
- Set up a business relationship with another massage therapist who has an established client base.
- Buy an existing massage therapy practice, or buy the physical assets of a practice.
- Expand by accepting insurance clients. (See "Pros and Cons of Seeking Third Party Reimbursement," chapter 3, figure 3.20, page 151.)

Moving to full-time status requires that you serve more clients, and might also include increasing the frequency of appointments with your existing clients.

Diversification

A massage practice can grow by selling more to its existing clients. You can do this by diversifying into new services and/or products. Clients who no longer have as much need for or interest in one service might make an appointment for something new. Likewise, the wider variety of services may attract new clients who are interested in one or more of the added offerings.

If you diversify your services with new massage modalities, be sure to share your new knowledge with your clients. Communicate this even if it is just a single thought or technique to add to what you already do. Clients may hear something they like and then be willing to try it. Use a variety of ways to let them know about your new diversified services:

- Provide marketing literature that details your background in massage, including the schools you have attended and for how many hours.
- Update your marketing literature as you continue your education. Hang new certificates on your wall.
- Send direct mail to clients.

Add Adjunct Therapies and Services

Similarly, many massage therapists offer adjunct therapies such as aromatherapy or facials. They may offer other services as well, such as yoga classes or reflexology. To add adjunct therapies, you should obtain additional training to provide them yourself, or you may engage others who have the qualifications to provide them. Be sure these adjunct therapies are consistent with the professional image of your practice.

Add Health-Related Products

Many massage therapists sell health-related products, from books and music to aromatherapy supplies, nutritional supplements, and essential oils. Be sure that the products you sell support the overall image you desire for your practice. Display the products attractively and be prepared to answer questions about them.

When you sell products, you may want to use some form of cross-selling. Cross-selling involves treating a mix of products and services as a package. For example, if you do neuromuscular massage for $60 per session and offer paraffin for the hands at $15, you could offer the two for a price of $67.50. Similarly, you might sell a facial pack with a massage. As your practice increases, you may find that some percentage of your clients like these packages. Experiment with different combinations to see what appeals most to clients.

Changing Specializations

As an established practitioner, you may decide to change the focus of your practice. This goal may result from a shift in clients' wants or needs. Or perhaps you simply have a desire to try something new or to become more specialized.

Your strategy to specialize will depend on whether you have decided to work with a specialized population and/or to develop specialized skills. An example of a specialized population is clients needing sports massage. When massage therapists decide to make the athlete population their focus, they take courses and workshops that will train them in this topic. Assuming you already have a base of clients, you probably would want to shift your focus in a way that gives you time to encourage your clients to try your new specialty or to refer them to another massage therapist.

Other examples of specialty fields include pregnancy or infant massage, geriatric massage, and animal massage. Perhaps you have a few clients in this group and you want to spend more time meeting their unique needs. Whatever focus you choose, however, be sure to get additional training to meet the specialized needs of your target market.

Pursuing Related Opportunities

Many massage therapists love learning and teaching. Their commitment to the profession of massage therapy may include a desire to advance knowledge of massage and its benefits. If your interests are in these areas, you may want to share or increase knowledge by becoming a teacher or researcher.

Becoming a Teacher

Some massage therapists advance their own learning so they can train others. Teaching is a satisfying activity in its own right, especially if you enjoy exercising your intellect and working with other professionals and students. Many massage therapists vary their routine by combining teaching with a massage therapy practice.

To become an approved provider of Category A continuing education, contact the National Certification Board for Therapeutic Massage and Bodywork (NCBTMB) at 1-800-296-0664. In addition, states that license massage therapists also may approve therapists as Continuing Education Unit providers. Contact the state's licensing agency to find out how to become listed. To teach at a massage school, contact the school's administrators to learn the qualifications required.

Born to Teach

Cynthia M. Ribeiro seems to have been born to teach, and to learn. After earning a degree in physical education, Ribeiro began to teach swimming, helping people deal with fears and physical disabilities. Eager to learn more about the human body, she also studied to become a nurse. Later, she moved from her birthplace, Brazil, to the United States to learn massage.

Ribeiro launched her career in massage therapy in Southern California, where she provided massages at a variety of sites, including hotels, chiropractors' offices, and an orthopedist's office. Her hotel clients were primarily interested in massage for relaxation. However, she naturally educated them in understanding the sources of whatever discomforts they reported. When her clients request relief from a particular problem, she counsels them to learn about their bodies and refers them to other professionals when appropriate.

Ribeiro has continued to live out her commitment to lifelong learning by actively seeking out opportunities for continuing education. Every year she takes several courses through AMTA and local training institutes.

The next step was almost inevitable: Ribeiro started a school, the Western Institute of Neuromuscular Therapy, in Laguna Hills, California. She cut back her private practice to teach and provide massages free to clients of the school. Although her hourly earnings from teaching do not match the income she received from giving massages, Ribeiro has no regrets about this phase of her career. She loves being in a learning environment and sharing her enthusiasm for the profession.

Source: Knaster, Mirka. "Cynthia Ribeiro: Help Your Clients to Reach Their Goals." *Massage Therapy Journal* (Summer 1998): 33-34, 36, 38.

When your practice is established, you naturally think about how to grow. The possibilities in the field of massage therapy are great, and they are increasing every day. Plan your growth so that it fits your goals. Whether you engage others, teach, or decide to increase your massage hours, be sure to nourish your personal growth and private life along with the size of your practice. Turn often to the reference sources and to your network of professional therapists. Coupled with your growing experience, these resources can enrich your understanding as well as increase your productivity.

Reevaluating Your Plan

If you followed all the steps in your "Career and Practice Plan" (chapter 2, figure 2.24, page 102), you will be prepared to evaluate your plan and your practice. Revisit that plan, and your initial hard work will help you with your next steps. Read each section of your plan, and ask questions about it. The questions in the "Plan Evaluation Worksheet" (figure 7.16, page 268) will help with that process. They will also help you plan how to keep your skills up-to-date.

If your plan differs from your career, you need to make changes. Perhaps you really like the way your practice has grown, even though it has not been according to plan. For example, maybe you were intimidated by the prospect of dealing with the medical establishment and thought you would avoid working closely with medical professionals. Now, however, you find yourself working closely with several MDs and DCs and enjoying it. In this case, you can change your plan, or rewrite it entirely if that suits you better. Literally take out the plan you prepared and update it by writing down your changes. This will help you visualize what you want to do and will keep your activities in line with your (new) goals.

In another situation, change might be necessary for you to make progress in carrying out your original plan. For example, if you do not have enough clients to meet expenses, you will need to get more. If you are not working in the modality that most interests you, you will have to develop a base of clients who want that modality. If you have too many clients, you will have to decide whether to cut back the number of clients you serve or bring in someone who can help you with those you have. Keep in mind that clients are seeing you because of your skills and your therapeutic relationship with them. If your client base is growing, it will probably be best to refer new clients to new practitioners who join you.

Or, you might find that you made changes to your plan but did not follow through on them. As a result of your review, you may discover a need to develop new strategies and tactics.

Of course, you may also see some areas in which you are right on target. If so, be sure to congratulate yourself. Continue to stop and be grateful for each small accomplishment on the way toward fulfilling your plans. Remember that your plan is a map of the territory, and a map is only one part of the whole. Taking a step back and getting a vision of the larger picture can help you refine your plans.

What Has Worked for You?

In revising your plans, consult the ideas in this and other books, and couple them with the wisdom of experience. Learn from your own experience and that of others you respect. If you have been keeping careful client records, you will have good information to help you decide what is working for you. Identify the different client types and/or modalities used in your practice. Then analyze them by answering the following questions:

- Which type of client gives you the best earnings per hour?
- Which provides the most repeat business?
- Which gives you the most satisfaction?
- Which do you want to focus on?
- Where did these clients come from? (For example, if they were referrals, from whom? If they were responses to advertising, where did they see the ads?)

As you grow your practice, focus on the activities (referrals, advertising, and so on) that are most effective in bringing you your target clients.

Figure 7.16   PLAN EVALUATION WORKSHEET

Reevaluating your business and marketing plans periodically is an important step that will help keep your practice healthy. Answer the following questions about your present business situation. If you decide to change any of your business objectives or activities, revise your Career and Practice Planning Worksheet to reflect your new plans.

1. Are your overall goals, as stated in the plan, still what you want to do? If not, what do you want to change?
   _____
   _____

2. Do you want to continue serving the same group of clients? If not, what client group do you want to target now? _____
   _____

3. Are you interested in providing the same kinds of services? If not, what do you want to change? _____
   _____
   _____

4. Are you interested in selling the same products (if any)? If not, what do you want to change? _____
   _____
   _____

5. Are your practice location and equipment appropriate and sufficient for your activities? If not, what do you want to change? _____
   _____

6. Is your staffing adequate and appropriate for meeting your objectives? If not, what do you want to change?
   _____
   _____

7. Are your financial objectives the same? If not, what are your new objectives? _____
   _____
   _____

8. Do your plans still seem attainable? If not, what changes are necessary? _____
   _____
   _____

9. Overall, based on your previous answers, are you on track to achieving your objectives? _____
   a. If so, what is working? _____
   b. If not, what needs to change? _____

the
BUSINESS
of MASSAGE

© 2002 American Massage Therapy Association, Evanston, IL. *The Business of Massage*. All Rights Reserved. #20026

What Has Worked for Others?

You can learn from other people's experience as well. Talk to other massage therapists about what they do to build their practices. Ask whether their ideas might apply to your practice. Seek advice from others who have successfully built a practice or business. Think creatively, and look for ways to apply lessons learned by business or practice owners in other fields, as well as your own.

Keep Your Skills Up-to-Date

As you review your practice's performance, look for ways to keep your skills current. Basic techniques for doing this are to maintain your credentials and to participate in continuing education. See chapter 8, "Connecting with the Professional Community," for more information about credentials and continuing education.

Recovery Strategies

It's the rare practice that starts out strong and continues to improve without encountering a major or minor downturn at some point. When it happens to you, it's important that you recognize the danger signs in time that you can do something about remedying the problems.

Red flags can be obvious or subtle. Subtle indicators of trouble could be the fact that the phone doesn't ring as often as it used to, or your general sense that clients aren't entirely satisfied after their sessions even if they don't voice a complaint.

The most obvious red flags are the number of clients you have booked each month, the amount of money you take in, and the level of expenses you pay out each month. Those three measurements are easy to keep track of, so you never have to be caught off-guard when your business encounters a decline. In setting up your business, you determined how many clients you would need per month in order to bring in the minimum level of income you would need, and the maximum level of expenses you could afford.

You might want to record these numbers on a tracking document, to make it easy to see trends that could spell trouble for the future health of your business. Highlight in yellow any indicators that fall outside the parameters of where they should be, and highlight in green the indicators that fall within your parameters. This gives you an easy visual indicator of the health of your business on a monthly basis—or make up a weekly tracking chart if you want to exert tighter control. See "At-a-Glance Health of Your Business" (figure 7.17, page 270) for a sample of what such a chart might look like.

Figure 7.17 At-a-Glance Health of Your Business

Month	# Clients (must be > ____)	Income (must be > $____)	Expenses (must be < $____)
January	_____	_____	_____
Feb	_____	_____	_____
March	_____	_____	_____
April	_____	_____	_____
Etc.	_____	_____	_____

When you see a trend that alerts you to trouble, you will want to analyze the factors that are causing that trend to occur. It's important to be realistic and accurate in identifying the underlying factors because clear identification will help you develop effective strategies for restoring your business to health.

It can be helpful to categorize factors according to those you can affect directly versus those that you can affect only indirectly. See "Recovery Strategies," (figure 7.18, page 271 for a summary of factors that could affect your business and related strategies that could help recover from business downturns.

Maintain Your Enthusiasm

Recognize when your business slumps that this is a normal cycle for almost every business. When it happens to you, it's important to analyze the factors that could be causing it so that you can take steps to bring it back to its former vitality. If massage therapy continues to be your chosen career path, don't be afraid to invest the time, energy, and creativity required to keep your career healthy.

Figure 7.18 Recovery Strategies

Factors and Recovery Actions

Factor	Your Actions Affect Directly/Indirectly	Possible Strategies
Local economy	Indirectly	Become involved with economic development in your community and propose ways to help stimulate the local economy.
Services/Modalities	Directly	Take training that will enable you to provide additional modalities, which will appeal to a broader target client audience. Announce through public relations or advertising channels that your practice now offers this new service and its associated benefits.
Marketing	Directly	Assess the effectiveness of your marketing plan. Are there cost-effective ways you can reach more prospective clients? Is your client retention plan effective? Can you educate a wider audience through public relations efforts?
Customer Service	Directly	Listen closely to your customer satisfaction feedback. Examine your incidence of repeat customers. Meet with your mentor or seek supervision to help identify how you can improve your service to and relationship with clients. See chapter 6 for more information.
Financial Management	Directly	Is your budget realistic? Are you exceeding your expenses and/or under-running your income? Your marketing plan will address how to attract more clients. Your examination of expenses will identify whether there are areas where you can reduce your expenses.

Chapter Summary

The purpose of a good marketing plan is to make your practice visible and attract clients to it. In developing your plan, you weigh the pros and cons of how to attract clients to your business, and you choose the ways that fit your goals and your budget. Your marketing plan consists of four parts: 1) goals, 2) objectives, 3) strategies, and 4) tactics.

Your target market, your budget, and where you are in your business cycle of growth influence the strategies you will choose. For instance, are you starting a new business and needing to attract all new clients, or do you want to expand an already existing practice? Strategies you might choose from include: personal selling (networking), advertising, public relations, sales promotions, and direct marketing.

Once you have selected appropriate strategies for your business, you will decide which tactics, or marketing practices, will be effective for you. These marketing practices could be carried out through print communications, electronic, or in person. Examples of print include brochures, business cards, gift certificates or coupons, and newsletters. Examples of electronic include Web sites and participation in electronic directories that let potential clients search for massage therapists by location or specialty. Personal selling tactics could include participation in networking and referrals to and from other healthcare professionals.

To determine whether your strategies and tactics continue to be appropriate for your business, you will need to reevaluate your plan on a regular basis. You might decide that you want to diversify your services or products, that you want to change your target market, or that you want to add insurance reimbursement clients. Depending on your desired changes, you would develop a current marketing plan that best supports your new goals.

Part of need for continual reevaluation of your business is to recognize danger signs that indicate a downturn. Danger signs could include fewer clients, client complaints, or rising expenses. The key to implementing a recovery strategy is identifying the problems early enough to fix them. By analyzing which problems are within your control and which aren't, you will be able to develop a revitalized marketing plan and recovery strategy that puts your business back on the road to good health.

Review Questions

1. What are the four primary parts of a marketing plan, and what is the purpose of each part?

2. Name at least three marketing strategies you can use to develop and maintain a client base.

3. Give at least one example of a tactic that would be appropriate for each type of marketing strategy.

4. What are the pros and cons of various marketing strategies?

5. What is the difference between a feature and a benefit?

6. What are some of the warning signals that your practice is experiencing a downturn?

7. What are examples of recovery strategies that could help your business if you experience a downturn?

8

CONNECTING *with* the PROFESSIONAL COMMUNITY

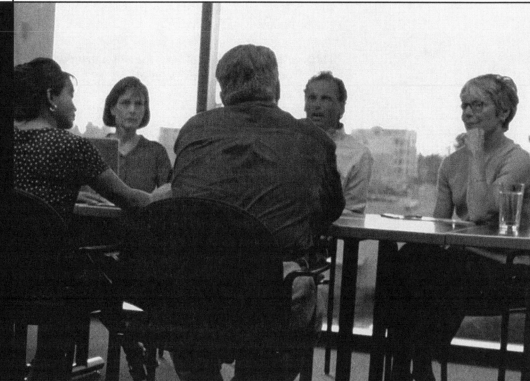

YOU'RE NOW A PART OF A WIDER COMMUNITY OF PROFESSIONALS WHO CARE JUST AS MUCH ABOUT MASSAGE THERAPY AS YOU DO.

Chapter Objectives

1. Identify agencies, professional associations, and other allied professions that massage practitioners commonly do business with.
2. Identify the role of professional associations for massage practitioners.
3. Identify strategies for effective communication with other professionals regarding client care and networking.
4. Identify strategies for conflict resolution in relationships with other professionals.
5. Identify characteristics of effective interaction in groups and organizations.
6. Identify strategies to attain new knowledge.
7. Demonstrate the ability to read and critically evaluate technical information found in health-related journals.
8. Explain the need for utilizing professional supervision when appropriate.

Your Place Within the Profession

You are, or soon will be, a member of the profession of massage therapy. It's a weightier statement than it might at first appear. Being a professional is both a privilege and a responsibility. This chapter explores the breadth of opportunities open to you. It will help you expand your presence within the profession and your value to it. Gaining your certificate or diploma from a well-respected program is, as you might suspect, the tip of the iceberg.

Being a professional opens the door to personal and career growth in many ways, and expands your opportunities to extend your skills and gifts to benefit of the greatest number of people.

Three primary components of professionalism are:
1. Your professional association
2. Continuing education
3. Research and advocacy

Your Professional Association

The role of a professional association in your personal and career development can be as limited or as encompassing as you choose to make it. At its most pragmatic, professional associations offer liability insurance for their members and members' clients' protection. A professional association not only supports your practice through member benefits but also helps advance the profession as a whole, with media, healthcare, and insurance professionals, legislative bodies, and the general public. At its fullest extent, a professional association offers the environment within which you join with other professionals to further the profession through advocacy, education, and research.

One of the foremost advantages of becoming actively involved in your professional association is that you have the opportunity to collaborate with your peers in the field of massage therapy. No one else understands the challenges, the frustrations, the deep satisfaction, and the inspirational visions for the profession as keenly as you and another peer. With your peers you can fashion strategies that keep the face of your profession turned toward the future in such a way that benefits you, your peers, your clients, and the public.

When choosing which professional association to join, ask the following questions about what each association offers:
1. *To what extent does it increase public awareness of the profession?*
   Does it conduct national public relations and marketing campaigns? Does it promote the profession through high visibility efforts such as AMTA's National Massage Therapy Awareness Week?
2. *Does it support massage research through the investment of time and money?*
   Does it provide leadership in establishing an agenda for massage research that will educate healthcare professionals on the benefits of massage and result in encouraging referral business from the medical community?

3. *Does it define and uphold ethics and standards for members?*
   Look at associations' history of development of ethics and standards for practitioners and schools in the area of certification and accreditation. Consider the rigor and peer review process required in the development and continued application of these standards.
4. *Does it foster legislative advocacy?*
   Consider to what extent it fosters a positive environment in which massage therapists can practice. Does it conduct ongoing contact with legislators and track legislation related to healing arts and complementary and alternative medicine so it can support its members' best interests?
5. *Is it member driven?*
   As a member, do you have a vote in what your association does to support the profession? Do you have the opportunity to influence change in the profession, in legislation, in the insurance industry, and in your professional association?
6. *What are its member benefits and the cost of membership?*
   In addition to its liability insurance coverage, what other benefits does the association offer? Many provide discounts on legal services, professional training, continuing education, conferences, massage therapy products and services, credit cards and other personal services. Does it publish a professional journal, and of what quality? Does it offer extensive opportunities for your personal involvement on a local, regional, and national level? Does it make it easy for you to participate with professional peers?

Many massage therapists maintain memberships in a national organization or association, such as American Massage Therapy Association, Associated Bodywork and Massage Professionals, or International Massage Association, and/or in an organization that serves a particular region or specialized modality or market. An example would be someone who is a member of AMTA and also a member of American Organization for Bodywork Therapies of Asia (AOBTA).

Promoting the Profession of Massage

Massage practitioners, like other professionals, are expected to establish and uphold standards for their profession, and to communicate those standards to others outside the profession. This increases clients' assurance that they will receive a high standard of care, which in turn benefits both you and your clients. The primary ways in which you promote your profession are through your individual behavior and through your involvement in organizations that extend the visibility of massage therapy in a positive light.

For example, as an individual you are professionally responsible to uphold your association's code of ethics and standards of practice. In addition, you promote the profession when you are enthusiastic and informative about your work. Massage practitioners can go even further in promoting the profession:
* They can actively participate in professional associations such as AMTA and events such as AMTA's National Massage Therapy Awareness Week (the last full week in October).

- They can write letters to government officials and support the development of massage therapy directed regulation that is fair for the profession.

Your efforts make a difference in helping influence the perceptions of massage held by legislators, healthcare specialists in other professions, and the public. In doing so, the profession of massage grows by attracting more clients and by enabling practitioners to be successful financially as well as in body, mind, and spirit. By investing a portion of your time and skills in supporting the profession that supports you, you are improving your work environment not only for yourself, but also for your peers and for those who follow in massage training.

Perspectives on Allied Professions

One aspect of being a professional is the interaction between members of your own profession, as discussed above. Another important aspect is the interaction with members of allied or related professions in a way that promotes cooperation and collaboration among members of the medical and complementary/alternative medicine professions.

One reason it's important to relate to members of allied professions, as well as within your own, is that you can be a spokesperson who builds bridges when differing perspectives arise. Many in the general public do not have a clear understanding of the relative merits of massage therapy (let alone the different modalities within this profession), physical therapy, chiropractic, osteopathy, naprapathy, naturopathy, homeopathy, acupuncture, and other professions. The same is true of professionals within each of those fields, and it's possible that you don't have any greater understanding of their profession than they do of yours. The more you interact with members of allied professions, the more opportunities you have to educate them and to learn about their professions from their perspectives.

Scope of Practice

Scope of practice is defined by whatever legal body has authority to specify the services a member of the profession may or may not perform. The legal authority will vary from jurisdiction to jurisdiction—it may be a state, a province, or a national government. States might impose more stringent rules than a national regulatory body, and municipalities more stringent than states, all levels of which practitioners are required to follow. To operate outside this scope would constitute a violation of law.

In addition to the legal scope of practice every practitioner must adhere to, every profession defines its own scope of practice. This is for the purpose of sharing a common language and understanding among peer professionals, but it does not take the place of the officially defined scope of practice that regulates practice in specific states, provinces, or municipalities.

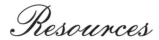

Where to Get Information About
Allied Professions

Note: This list is not intended to be exhaustive, but it contains contact information for some of the professions with which you might come into contact.

- American Chiropractic Association (ACA), 1701 Clarendon Blvd., Arlington, VA 22209; (800) 986-4636; www.amerchiro.org
- American Occupational Therapy Association (AOTA), 4720 Montgomery Lane, Bethesda, MD 20824-1220; (301) 652-2682; www.aota.org
- American Osteopathic Association (AOA), 142 East Ontario Street, Chicago, IL 60611; (800) 621-1773 or (312) 202-8000; www.aoa-net.org
- American Fitness Professionals & Associates (AFPA), P.O. Box 214, Ship Bottom, NJ 08008; (609) 978-7583; www.afpafitness.com
- American Physical Therapy Association (APTA), 1111 N. Fairfax Street, Alexandria, VA 22314-1488; 800-999-APTA; www.apta.org
- Canadian Chiropractic Association (CCA), 1396 Eglinton Ave. West Toronto ON M6C 2E4; www.ccachiro.org
- Canadian College of Osteopathy (CCO), 39 Alvin Avenue, Toronto, Ontario, Canada M4T 2A7; (416) 323-1465; www.osteopathy-canada.com
- Canadian Massage Therapist Alliance (CMTA), 365 Bloor Street East, Suite 1807, Toronto, Ontario, Canada M4W 3L4; (416) 968-2149; www.collinscan.com:8099/CMTA/cmtai.html
- Canadian Medical Association (CMA), 1867 Alta Vista Drive, Ottawa, ON, Canada K1G 3Y6, 613-731-9331; www.cma.ca
- Canadian Naturopathic Association (CNA), 1255 Sheppard Avenue East, North York, Ontario, Canada M2K 1E2; (416) 496-8633; www.naturopathicassoc.ca
- Canadian Touch Research Center (CTRC), 760, Saint-Zotique Street East, Montreal, Quebec, Canada H2S 1M5; (514) 272-2254; www.ccrt-ctrc.org
- International SPA Association (ISPA), 2365 Harrodsburg Rd., Suite A325, Lexington, KY 40504; (859) 226-4372; www.experienceispa.com
- National Athletic Trainers' Association (NATA), 2952 Stemmons Freeway, Dallas, Texas 75247-6916; (800).TRY.NATA (800-879-6282); www.nata.org
- National Strength and Conditioning Association (NSCA), 1955 N. Union Blvd., Colorado Springs, CO 80909; (719) 632-6722 or (800) 815-6826; www.nsca-lift.org

In most jurisdictions, a massage practitioner is not allowed to "treat," "diagnose," or "prescribe." However, massage therapists are allowed to practice certain services in some states that other states prohibit. For instance, the state of Florida allows massage therapists to perform ultrasound; the state of Maryland does not. It is important that you understand the scope of practice defined by your state or province. It would contribute to your professional breadth of understanding, if you were to be knowledgeable about the scopes of practices of other allied professions in your state as well.

Every massage therapist has a personal responsibility to practice only to the extent of his or her education, training and qualifications, regardless of scope of practice. An experienced massage therapist will undoubtedly practice a wider range of services, still within the given scope, than will an entry level practitioner.

Building Bridges Between Professions

You will want to communicate professionally and to establish networking relationships that mutually benefit you and your allied peers. Therefore, you will want to have a basic understanding of each profession's scope of practice (which may vary from state to state), the profession's basic concepts of practice, and its members' level of professional training. Just as it is important for you to know how many hours of training a particular specialist is required to have, it is important that you educate your professional counterparts about how many hours of massages you have provided, in addition to your core training.

A key to communicating effectively with members of allied professions is in understanding the other specialist's terminology and depth of training. For example, the term "range of motion" can be the basis for honest miscommunication between a massage practitioner and a physical therapist (PT). As a massage practitioner, you might tell a physical therapist that you can be helpful to a client in increasing his or her range of motion. To you, this means you can increase the mobility of a client's limb to a greater range than the client could move it before having a session with you. To a PT, however, range of motion refers to an entire area of study in which the PT has a very extensive level of knowledge and training.

Another example is comparing how a massage practitioner, a physical therapist, and a chiropractor use the term "PNF" (proprioceptive neuromuscular facilitation). The massage practitioner has a basic understanding of PNF, and is probably trained in one or several contract-and-relax techniques that would be acceptably classified as PNF techniques. The PT and chiropractor, however, have undergone training in which PNF is studied as an entire complex system and in which they are trained to apply specific and sometimes sophisticated treatments to aid the client. For a massage practitioner to assume that PNF means the same thing to all specialists would lead the PT to believe that the massage practitioner is not knowledgeable about the level of training required by a PT.

Resolving Conflict

A misunderstanding between professionals can be remedied if both parties focus on the similarities rather than on the differences between them, and recognize the fact that they both want to achieve the same thing: a more healthful outcome for the client.

Approach a dialogue with a peer professional from the point of view of wanting to clarify what he or she is communicating to you. As in the examples of "range of motion" and "PNF" above, sincere dialogue about what each person means by this terminology will go a long way toward fostering appreciation of the other specialist's intent.

The basic goal in establishing productive working relationships that enhance the perception and quality of each other's work is to develop a genuine appreciation for what another specialist's strengths are. You can enhance each other's professional image by understanding how your two professions complement each other. For instance, many chiropractors appreciate the increased mobility a massage can give a client, which can allow the client's chiropractic session to be more effective than it might have been without a prior massage.

Be aware that you might encounter overlapping areas of work between your scopes of practice. When this is the case, simply acknowledge that although some services or techniques may be common to both professions, a practitioner of one or the other profession is probably specifically qualified to a greater or lesser degree than the other to help a client in a particular way.

When you know you will be talking with a member of an allied profession, it would be helpful if you had with you written educational materials about the efficacy of massage that you could share. Another way you can educate members of allied professions is to offer to present educational sessions to their colleagues and staff. This could either be in the format of a prepared speech (see chapter 7) or in an informal discussion in the office lunchroom. Your willingness to share information that could benefit clients and members of allied professions, and your knowledge of the benefits of massage, will aid you as well as the entire profession of massage therapy.

Continuing Education

Ongoing education is essential to professional growth. The organizations through which you are licensed and nationally certified, and of which you are a member, have continuing education requirements for maintaining your credentials or membership status. See "Requirements for Nationally Certified Massage Therapists and Bodyworkers" on page 282.

Education can be for the purpose of refreshing skills you know already or learning new ones. You might decide to expand your knowledge in-depth by taking as much additional training as you can in a given specialty area. Or you might find that expanding your breadth of training—taking continuing education sessions in a variety of topics—is more suitable for you. NCBTMB requires that renewing practitioners take at least two hours of ethics continuing education every four years.

Strategies for Attaining New Knowledge

There is formal training and informal training. Your strategy for attaining new knowledge through either of these methods will be different. Formal training is what you need to earn the continuing education credits required for you to maintain your professional credentials or membership status. Informal is the method through which you greet every experience as an opportunity to attain new knowledge.

Formal Training

A good time to devise a game plan for taking continuing education is when you reevaluate your business plan and when you prepare your annual expense budget. Evaluating your business plan prompts you to review your long-term goals and to set new directions for your career or business. If you have employees, you should include continuing education objectives as part of your expectations as an employer. Remember, your objectives for upgrading your skills— and the services you offer—should support your overall business goals.

Depending on your goals, you may decide to take training in a new modality, to change your career direction, or to acquire more in-depth knowledge in a specialty area you already practice. By looking at least a year in advance, you can plan ahead for the expense involved and include it in your budget.

Planning ahead enables you to make the most of your upcoming training by reading related materials prior to attending a class or workshop. Then, when you are in the presence of an instructor/specialist, you will have the opportunity to ask questions about areas of the topic that might go into more depth than what is presented during class.

Also, by planning ahead you have the chance to combine your continuing education goals with your personal goals. If you want to take a spring vacation to a certain area of the country, you might research which schools of massage or chapters of professional associations are in that part of the country, and time your vacation with continuing education opportunities. Combining your education and vacation plans also helps you stretch your budget dollars further.

Informal Training

Informal training is one of the self-care benefits you can build into your routine every day. Opportunities for continual knowledge attainment abound when you approach the world with an inquiring mind. Every massage session, if you focus your observation skills, gives you information about the effectiveness of your touch techniques on the client. Every conversation with a client offers new opportunities for you to refine your communications and customer service skills. Conversations with peers or other professionals introduce topics that you might want to research further.

You might want to "formalize" informal training by scheduling 30 minutes a day specifically for knowledge attainment. This could consist of reading a journal, listening to a tape, watching a video, and reading information on Web sites. You might want to assign yourself a "topic of the month" and learn as much as you can about a particular modality.

At the end of every day, get in the habit of asking yourself, "What new thing did I learn today?" and "What do I want to learn tomorrow?"

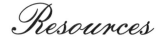

Where to Find Continuing Education
- massage schools
- community colleges
- AMTA's continuing education calendar: www.amtamassage.org
- *Massage Therapy Journal* advertising
- *Massage Magazine* advertising
- NCBTMB's continuing education provider listings: www.ncbtmb.com
- research institutes

Requirements for Nationally Certified Massage Therapists and Bodyworkers

The National Certification Board for Therapeutic Massage and Bodywork (NCBTMB) establishes specific requirements for achieving and maintaining national certification. The following requirements are necessary to become Nationally Certified:

- You must graduate from a minimum 500-hour in-class, formal training program. If you have not completed a 500 hour in-class, formal training program, you must satisfy the requirements set forth in the Portfolio Review Handbook.

- You must submit documentation, including an official transcript, a notarized copy of diploma, or a notarized certificate of completion.

- You must submit a complete application with the appropriate fee.

- You must pass the National Certification Exam (NCE).

In order to recertify, every four years you must demonstrate 200 hours of work experience, submit a completed application with appropriate fee and either pass the current form of the NCE or demonstrate 50 hours of continuing education. Below are the criteria for meeting the continuing education requirements:

- At least twenty-five hours of continuing education must be conducted by NCBTMB Category A Approved Providers and meet NCBTMB criteria.

- No more than twenty-five hours may be in Category B (other continuing education that meets NCBTMB's definition of continuing education).

- Two hours of the continuing education must be on the topic of professional ethics.

- You may get continuing education credit for up to five hours of teaching and up to five hours of writing published articles.

- Continuing education may include conferences, short courses, seminars, workshops, or home study programs.

For further details and up-to-date requirements, consult the NCBTMB Recertification Handbook or contact NCBTMB (1-800-296-0664). Information may also be obtained on the Web site at www.ncbtmb.com.

Research

The volume and importance of research in the field of massage therapy has grown in recent years. Not only do experienced massage therapists enjoy contributing to the growing body of research into the benefits of massage, but the opportunities and funding to do so have increased. It is only recently that the public has turned to more nontraditional forms of health care and wellness, that massage has become more popular. This has led to questions about the use, safety, and efficacy of massage by healthcare professionals in the allopathic, or medical, community, which in turn has contributed to the increase in research on massage.

Increased Opportunities for Research

Momentum has built since 1999 that bodes well for the availability of increased research in massage therapy. One example is that the National Center for Complementary and Alternative Medicine (NCCAM) of the National Institutes of Health (NIH) committed $68.4 million to CAM research. Another is that the AMTA Foundation convened the Massage Research Agenda Workgroup (MRAW), which identified specific areas of study and goals for massage therapy research. One of the observations a group of massage therapy professionals and research scientists who comprised the MRAW made was that there are a lot of claims about the benefits of massage therapy but not much research. For more information about the MRAW, see the AMTA Foundation Web site (www.amta-massage.org/foundation).

A third example of increased emphasis on research is that the AMTA Foundation developed the Massage Therapy Research Database^{SM}, a listing of articles on massage therapy research. This database makes accessing research studies about massage free, and convenient to anyone who visits the AMTA Foundation Web site.

Another step that occurred in late 2001 was that AMTA, the AMTA Foundation, and Commission on Massage Therapy Accreditation (COMTA) participated in the "National Policy Dialogue for Integrative Health Care: Finding Common Ground." The results of this dialogue were presented to the White House Commission on Complementary and Alternative Medicine Policy. This was significant in that it was the first time leaders from so many CAM practices convened and searched for common ground so that policy could be recommended for a truly integrative healthcare system.

In "A New Era for Massage Research" [*Massage Therapy Journal*, Fall 2001, pages 104-114], author Janet Kahn cites the following reasons for pursuing massage therapy research:

1. Research—"the continual generation of a relevant body of knowledge"—is key to the professionalization of any healthcare field.
2. Research opens the doorway to those who desire to practice massage therapy in medical contexts, or who desire to be reimbursed by insurance. Insurance, in turn, makes massage therapy available to those who cannot now afford it.

The need for research becomes particularly apparent in light of the fact that the Agency for Health Care Quality and Research (AHCQR), a part of the U.S. Department of Health and Human Services, decides which services and treatments will be reimbursed for people whose health care is paid by Medicaid and Medicare. Agencies such as this one require credible scientific research in order to justify approving certain services for coverage. Agencies such as AHCQR make their decisions on the basis of published large, randomized control, double-blind and placebo-based studies that clearly show efficacy, safety, and cost-effectiveness of treatment modalities.

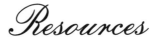

Organizations That Fund Massage Research
- AMTA Foundation, 820 Davis Street, Suite 100, Evanston, IL 60201, (847) 869-5019; www.amtamassage.org/foundation/home.htm
- Canadian Touch Research Center (CTRC), 760 St-Zotique Street East, Montreal, Canada H2S 1M5; 1-800-619-5463; real.gaboriault@ccrt-ctrc.org; www.ccrt-ctrc.org
- National Center for Complementary and Alternative Medicine, P.O. Box 8218, Silver Spring, MD 20907-8218, (888) 644-6226; www.altmed.od.nih.gov/nccam/
- Touch Research Institutes, University of Miami, School of Medicine, Dept. of Pediatrics, P.O. Box 016820, Miami, FL 33101; (305) 243-6781; e-mail: tfield@mednet.med.miami.edu; www.miami.edu/touch-research

What Topics Are Researched?
Research can help answer questions that lead to better understanding of how massage can improve people's lives. For example: Why or how does massage help premature infants gain more weight when they are massaged versus when they are not? How does self-healing occur? What is the role of a massage therapist in helping a client achieve peak performance?

These are just a few of the unanswered questions that point to the need for research in the field of massage therapy. Massage practitioners want to see research in topics that will help them communicate more information to clients and that will help them expand their practices. In the AMTA 2000 Segmentation Study, 96 percent of respondents said they wanted to be able to access research information for the following reasons:
- to improve their skills as therapists
- to help start or grow their practice
- to validate the medical benefits of massage
- to validate the mind/body benefits of massage
- to validate acceptance of the massage therapist as a professional

The MRAW identified qualities that describe conditions for a good massage research study topic, most of which can be applied to the areas shown above (see "Qualities of a Good Massage Research Study," below). Organizations that fund research can help you formulate a research project and proposal that could shed new light on any of these topics.

Qualities of a Good Massage Research Study

The Massage Therapy Research Agenda Workgroup
- Greater potential to alleviate human suffering or associated costs
- Affects many people's lives
- Usual treatment unacceptable in some way
- Study subjects readily available
- Expectation that massage therapy will be beneficial based on strong anecdotal evidence or pilot data
- Treatment should be easy to adopt
- Study must have clear massage therapy intervention
- Endpoints to be measured should be well-defined and important to stakeholders

Source: Janet R. Kahn. "A New Era for Massage Research." *Massage Therapy Journal*, Fall 2001, pages 104-114.

How to Participate in Research

To participate in research efforts, you can start by contacting organizations that sponsor research and inquiring about the opportunities available.

A good place to begin is with the AMTA Foundation. Since 1990, the AMTA Foundation has sponsored scholarships and community outreach, as well as research projects related to the efficacy of massage. Some of the studies sponsored by the AMTA Foundation have explored the effect of massage in caring for clients with migraine headaches, academic stress, grief, spinal cord injuries, and pain associated with sickle cell anemia and cancer. The AMTA Foundation also educates massage therapists about the research it sponsors, as well as about the basics of designing, conducting, and interpreting scientific research.

Other organizations that sponsor research about massage include the Bodywork Research Institute, the Touch Research Institutes (at the University of Miami School of Medicine), and the National Center for Complementary and Alternative Medicine. See "Resources: Organizations that Fund Massage Research" (page 284).

Many Ways to Become Involved in Massage Therapy Research

1. *Take a course on research methods.* Many colleges and universities offer courses on research methodology and statistics. Workshops have been held at AMTA national conventions.
2. *Review research that has been done.* Look at the sources listed in "Resources: Organizations that Fund Massage Research" (page 284) to access the latest information. Reviewing what research has been done may lead to new research questions. This may also lead to questions of the mechanisms of how massage works; new potential uses or interventions for massage; how massage may interface with other allied healthcare modalities; etc.
3. *Learn how to put together a good research proposal.* One source of helpful information is the AMTA Foundation Web site (www.amtamassage.org/foundation/home.htm). Go to "Research" to read informative articles by Martha Brown Menard, Ph.D., about how to develop your research questions.
4. *Find out deadlines for research application proposals and submit your proposal.*

Shared Wisdom

"If you wish to get involved in research, you should contact your local hospitals, local research centers, colleges and universities, and/or key practitioners in your geographic area. Read the newest studies and see if any are being done in your area. You could perhaps do a small study within your practice—be in touch with the AMTA Foundation about how to do this."

—*John Balletto, President, AMTA Foundation*

Identifying Biases in Research

It is very difficult to conduct a study that is totally objective, devoid of all tendencies to produce a result that proves what the researcher already suspects. That is why adherence to accepted research methods is so important. If you take a course in research methods and you become conversant with the factors that affect a study's validity, you will start to read the results critically. It is possible, in a study that is not conducted according to accepted research methods, for biases to be introduced, possibly without the researcher's knowledge or intent. Questions to determine the validity of research results include:

- Was the sample size of the study large enough from which to draw valid conclusions?
- How were the sample participants chosen?
- Did the study participants know the source of the study's funding?
- Was there a control group?
- What level and quality of statistical analysis was performed?
- Did the funding for the study come from a commercial source that might have unintentionally introduced a bias?
- Have the results been replicated by other scientists?
- Would it be possible for another scientist to replicate the results?

Suggesting that you be alert to biases does not mean that you view research negatively, but only that you view the results of a study with an accurate understanding of how they were achieved.

See "Five Steps to Getting the Most Out of Research Articles" (page 288) for helpful tips about how to read and evaluate research.

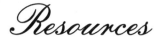

Articles about Research

- Bass, M., E. Dunn, P. Norton, M. Stewart, and F. Tudiver, (Eds.). *Conducting Research in the Practice Setting.* Newbury Park: Sage Publications, Inc., 1993.
- Bausell, R.B. *Conducting Meaningful Experiments: 40 Steps to Becoming a Scientist.* Thousand Oaks, California: Sage Publications, 1994.
- Cook, T.D., and Campbell, D.T. *Quasi-Experimentation: Design and Analysis Issues for Field Settings.* Boston: Houghton Mifflin, 1979.
- Hammell, K W, C. Carpenter, and I. Dyck, I. *Using Qualitative Research—A Practical Introduction for Occupational and Physical Therapists.* St. Louis, Missouri: W.B. Saunders Publications, Inc., 2000.
- Hammerly, Milt. *Responses to the White House Commission on Complementary and Alternative Medicine Policy.* December 5, 2000; Session VI: "CAM Integration in Delivery Systems."
- Harvey, Michael. "5 Steps to Getting the Most from Research Articles." *Massage Magazine*, March/April 2001, pages 165-166, 168-172.
- Jonas, Wayne B. "The Evidence House: How to Build an Inclusive Base for Complementary Medicine." *Western Journal of Medicine*, 2001: 175, pages 79-80.
- Krathwohl, David R. *Methods of Educational and Social Science Research.* New York: Longman Publishing Group, 1993.
- Krathwohl, David R. *How to Prepare a Research Proposal.* Syracuse: Syracuse University Press, 1988.
- Kuhn, T. *The Structure of Scientific Revolution.* Chicago: University of Chicago Press, 1970.
- Lincoln, Y.L., and E. G. Guba. *Naturalistic Inquiry.* Newbury Park: Sage Publications, Inc.,1985.
- Menard, Martha Brown. "An Introduction to Research Design." *Massage Therapy Journal*, Summer 1995.
- Menard, Martha Brown. *Making Sense of Research: A Guide to Research Literacy for Complementary Practitioners.* Toronto: Curties-Overzet Publications, Inc., 2002 (planned).
- Menard, Martha Brown. "How To Develop Your Research Question." *Massage Therapy Journal*, Winter 1996.
- Menard, Martha Brown. "An Introduction to Research Methods for Massage Therapists." *Massage Therapy Journal*, Summer 1994.
- Patton, M.Q. *Qualitative Evolution and Research Methods.* Newbury Park: Sage Publications, Inc., 1990.
- Ries, J., and C. Keukefeld, C. *Applying for Research Funding* Thousand Oaks, California: Sage Publications, Inc., 1995.

Five Steps to Get the Most Out of Research Articles

Step 1: Find the article
A few good places to look for research about massage are listed below:
* Alternative Therapies in Health and Medicine: www.alternative-therapies.com
* American Massage Therapy Association: www.amtamassage.org—click on Massage Information Center
* AMTA Foundation Massage Therapy Research Database℠: www.amtamassage.org/foundation
* Cochrane Library: www.update-software.com/ccweb/cochrane/revabstr/ccabout.htm
* MANTIS (Manual, Alternative and Natural Therapy): www.healthindex.com/MANTIS.asp
* National Center for Complementary and Alternative Medicine: www.nccam.nih.gov
* PubMed: http://igm.nlm.nih.gov (This site overlaps areas of Medline, the National Library of Medicine's database of healthcare literature.)
* Touch Research Institutes: www.miami.edu/touch-research
* University Web sites
* Do a general search on "massage therapy research" and "touch research."

Step 2: Prepare your mind
Prepare your mind to acquire new information. Realize that you are about to read a few pages where the author has packed a lot of information into each sentence. The information is usually cumulative, meaning that every paragraph builds upon the previous one. Take your time, and reread if you get distracted.

Step 3: Read the abstract
Most articles have an abstract or summary at the beginning or the end. Read that first. Also read the background section. If it's not labeled "background," look for discussion information just before the methods section.

Step 4: Read or skim the methods section
This is where the authors explain what they did and how they did it. This is where the author presents enough detail that another researcher could replicate the experiment accurately.

Step 5: Read or skim the results section
This section describes in detail how the data were collected and handled, as well as the analysis, recommendations for future studies, and/or therapeutic implications of the data. Don't become frustrated if you feel out of your element in the mathematical information; focus on the relevant findings as summarized in the abstract, the summary, or the discussion section.

Adapted from: Michael Harvey. "5 Steps to Getting the Most from Research Articles." *Massage Magazine*, March/April 2001, pp. 165-166, 168-172. Used by permission.

Glossary of Research Terms

ANOVA (analysis of variance): Statistical method that determines the effect of a test factor (such as a 15-minute massage) on a response variable (such as systolic blood pressure). ANOVA analyzes variability between groups, relative to the effects, and determines whether groups of data are similar, or different. This tool helps weed out differences due to normal variation from those actually produced by the independent variables.

blinding: Performed or made without the benefit of background information that might prejudice the outcome or result, e.g., blind taste tests used in marketing studies.

empirical: A method of inquiry that relies on subjects' experience or observation.

experimental group: Subjects who are receiving the trial intervention.

mean, m or x: The average. You can calculate the mean by adding all of the values and dividing by n (the sample size).

median: An indicator of the middle. Half of all observed values are above the median and half are below.

n: The sample size. If, for example, 20 individuals were evaluated, then n=20.

objective (adjective)*:* Information gathered by the use of measurement tools.

p-value: When perfoming a T-test (see below), a resultant p-value tells us how confident we can be in the result. Often we see the p-value <0.05 (or less than 5 percent). A T-test result might indicate that the means are different with a p-value of <0.05. This means that there's a 5 percent chance that the means are really the same and 95 percent confidence that the means are truly different.

placebo: A substance, technique, or protocol having no pharmacological effect but given to a patient or subject of an experiment who supposes it to be a medicine.

randomized: A research design in which subjects are arbitrarily placed in either the control group or experimental group.

standard deviation, SD or ±: how variable the data are about the mean. The symbol ± means, literally, plus or minus.

statistical significance: A method of analyzing data that demonstrates that there is a less than 5 percent chance that the finding occurred by chance. In other words, if something is statistically significant, there are five chances in 100 that the outcome was a fluke. And therefore, a 95 percent chance that the finding was not an accident.

subjective: Information reported by the subject.

T-test: Compares two means to determine whether they are statistically different from one another. The T-test will produce a p-value that will tell you how confident you can be in a result.

For example, when $p<0.05$, and the T-test indicates that the means are different, you can be 95 percent confident that the means are different as opposed to merely appearing different. Researchers know that sometimes things that look different may actually be the same—or more accurately, may have been sampled from the same pool—and only appear different to the naked eye. A good example would be something like body temperature or blood pressure. These vital signs vary within an individual as well as between individuals. Good use of ANOVA and a T-test will indicate whether apparent differences are real or simply due to natural variation.

trend: Data that lean toward a certain outcome, but are not statistically significant.

The Terms in Action
This fictitious example shows how some of the terms above are used. Consider the following pre-massage systolic blood pressures (mm Hg, or millimeters mercury, the units used in a standard blood pressure measurement):

118, 142, 108, 110, 158, 162, 104

Since there are seven blood-pressure measurements, n=7. The mean is 128.8. The median is 118, as there are three values below 118 (104, 108 and 110) and three values above 118 (142, 158, and 162).

A T-test might be used to measure systolic blood pressure prior to and following massage, for example. In this case, the mean values for each time point (the mean systolic blood pressure before massage and after massage) would be calculated, and then the means would be compared.

ANOVA used in a well-constructed study will help answer the question, "Was blood pressure really lowered after massage or did it simply go down because the test subjects laid still for 50 minutes?" and "If massage does affect blood pressure, how much?"

Adapted from "5 Steps to Getting the Most from Research Articles," by Michael Harvey. *Massage Magazine*, March/April 2001, pages 165-166, 168-172.

Professional Growth Through Supervision

Many massage therapists find they need someone to help them sort out the behaviors and feelings they experience while interacting with clients. They get this help from supervision—that is, a process of learning by discussing work experiences with peers or a more experienced therapist.

Massage therapists can use any of three kinds of supervision:
1. School clinic supervisor—This type of supervision usually focuses on the notes written after the student/client session. It may or may not be technique related. These supervisors help students understand where the students need to develop, or grow.
2. Group supervision—This involves a group of massage therapists coming together to talk through client issues they are experiencing. The therapists offer advice to each other based on their own experiences.
3. Professional supervision—A trained mental health professional who knows the theory of client-therapist relationships acts as a guide through a massage therapist's self-examination of professional issues. Ideally, a professional supervisor is trained in massage and the relationship issues it can bring out.

Because of the confidential nature of massage, the actual supervision is done outside the session. Supervision can help with many of the client issues that massage therapists encounter, from client hygiene or lack of cooperation, to a therapist's anger or other feelings aroused by a client's behavior. The supervisor also can help the massage therapist address particular issues related to specific client types. Supervision issues may fall into three categories:
1. the client-therapist relationship
2. what is occurring with the client psychologically and physically
3. what is occurring with the massage therapist psychologically and physically

Supervisors who have more experience can provide options for how a massage therapist can handle a situation the next time it arises.

When you are looking for a supervisor, keep in mind that different states have different qualifications for supervision. For example, Oregon's mental health board keeps a list of professional supervisors from the mental health field who are certified by the state. Check with your state board for such a list, or look for a counselor who is trained in massage. Also, note that the expense of paying for a supervisor generally is tax deductible.

Chapter Summary

Many massage therapists consider professional development to be among their highest priorities. To extend your time and energy to professional growth beyond your skills as an employee or business owner, you enhance your individual experience as well as contribute to the entire profession. Three areas that offer rich and satisfying opportunities for professional growth include joining a professional association, taking continuing education, and supporting research.

Your professional association offers many opportunities in addition to professional liability insurance. When selecting which professional association you will join, consider their contribution to the profession in terms of media exposure, legislative advocacy, quality of continuing education, opportunities to collaborate with your peers, and promoting massage to the general public and to allied professions.

You can build bridges with massage therapy's allied professions, such as chiropractic and physical therapy, as an individual as well. Relating positively to other professionals allows you to expand your business, as well as build productive alliances and extend your knowledge. By learning about the scope of your allied professionals' training and understanding the basics of their terminology, you will be able to educate them effectively about how massage therapy complements their clients' wellness or rehabilitation needs.

Another way in which to enhance your profession is to participate actively in continuing education opportunities. A specified number of continuing education credits over a given period of time are mandated by many professional organizations in the United States and Canada as a requirement of maintaining professional status as a member. Learning takes place in formal settings, such as classes and workshops, as well as informally. Adopting an attitude that views everyday experiences as learning opportunities allows you to expand your knowledge and your perceptions far beyond the classroom experience.

One area of continuing education that has become more important in recent years is massage therapy research. Massage therapists have indicated their hope that additional research about the efficacy of massage will help them improve their skills, validate the medical and body/mind benefits of massage, and help expand the acceptance of massage therapists as professionals. As a massage therapist, you may want to become involved in conducting or participating in research, or as a reader of massage therapy research that you can apply to the benefit of your business. Opportunities for both are growing rapidly.

Another area of professional development that many massage therapists find valuable is using a practice called supervision. Engaging the assistance of a professional supervisor allows you to sort out the behaviors and feelings you experience while interacting with clients. You would work with individual or group support, with experienced supervisors who can help you reflect on your experiences with clients. Feedback from a supervisor can help you enhance your therapeutic relationship with clients, improve your self-care, and improve the health of your business.

Growing as a professional within your own community of peers, community-wide, association chapter-wide, nationwide and worldwide, allows you to communicate how much you care about the massage therapy profession. An immense potential exists for extending the benefits of massage by focusing on the good of all, which includes the public, healthcare professionals, and your peers. Professional growth will make your career that much more rewarding.

Review Questions

1. What are major benefits of membership in a professional association for massage therapists?

2. Name examples of allied professions with which massage therapists commonly collaborate in order to extend their wellness benefits to patients.

3. When building relationships with members of allied professions, what communication skills can you apply regarding client care and networking?

4. What communication strategies can you use if your relationship with other professionals requires conflict resolution?

5. Identify strategies to attain new knowledge.

6. What skills are required in order to read and critically evaluate technical information found in health-related journals?

7. How would a massage therapist benefit from using professional supervision?

INDEX